A MARSHALL HEALTH GUIDE

# HERBAL REMEDIES

A MARSHALL HEALTH GUIDE

# HERBAL REMEDIES

The complete guide to the therapeutic herbal
relief of tension, stress, aches and pains

TAMARA KIRCHER
JADE BRITTON, MNIMH

MARSHALL PUBLISHING · LONDON

A QUARTO BOOK

First published in the UK in 1998 by
Marshall Publishing Ltd
170 Piccadilly
London W1V 9DD

ISBN 1–84028–071–9

This book was designed and produced by
Quarto Publishing plc
The Old Brewery
6 Blundell Street
London N7 9BH

Senior Art Editor: Elizabeth Healey
Editor: Judith Evans
Designer: Caroline Hill
Photographer: Bruce Mackie
Illustrator: Kevin Maddison
Picture Researcher: Zoë Holtermann
Indexer: Dorothy Frame
Managing Editor: Sally MacEachern
Editorial Director: Pippa Rubinstein
Assistant Art Director: Penny Cobb
Art Director: Moira Clinch

Typeset in Great Britain by
Central Southern Typesetters, Eastbourne
Manufactured in Singapore by
Bright Arts (Singapore) Pte. Ltd.
Printed in China by
Leefung-Asco Printers Ltd.

This book is not intended as a substitute for
the advice of a health care professional. The
reader should regularly consult a health
practitioner in matters relating to health,
particularly with respect to symptoms that
may require diagnosis or medical attention.

# CONTENTS

# FOREWORD

We are living in a time of great diversity, change and confusion. We are overwhelmed with choices of healing systems, concepts and treatment techniques. Some feel that herbal medicine is just one of a variety of alternative therapies. It is far from that, since it is used by up to 80 per cent of the world's population for their health care needs. Herbal medicine does not oppose conventional medicine, but can be used as first line therapy in a more natural healing fashion. In fact, many of today's modern or 'miracle' drugs have grown from the roots of herbalism. Even though modern medicine has its basis in herbalism, often a drug is over-refined and may lose some of the other components that complement or prevent side effects.

Plant medicine has been used in a therapeutic fashion since antiquity in the healing of body, mind and spirit. This philosophy is our heritage. Herbal medicine uses a holistic approach to healing and shows ways of life enhancement, rather than just

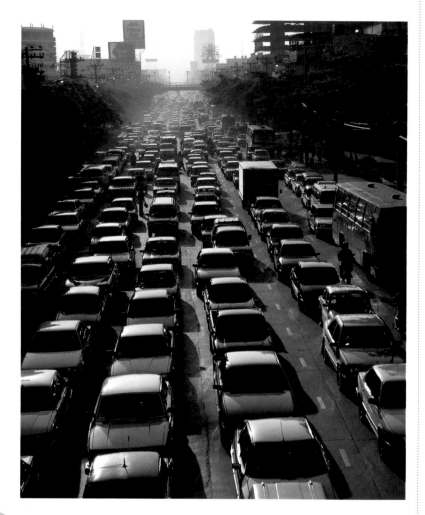

*Pollution caused by our consumer-driven society is threatening our health and the health of the planet as a whole.*

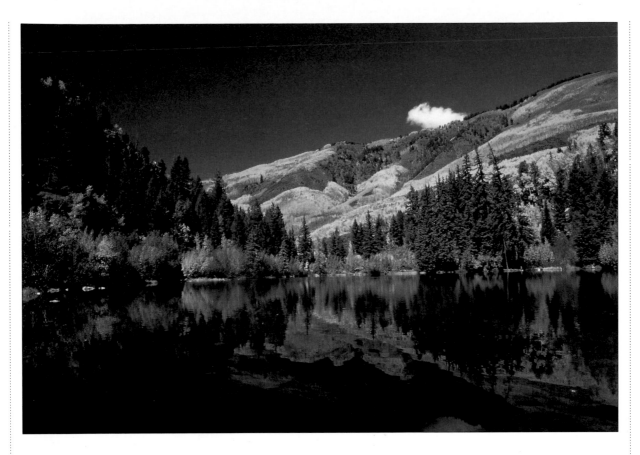

treating symptoms. Symptoms are our body's way of signalling that something is wrong and needs attention. By choosing natural methods, we choose to become more aware, connected and conscious.

This is a time of limited financial medical resources, and restricted availability of medical care. Herbal medicine is in the perfect position to fill the gap and treat both simple and complicated medical problems. Although the theory of herbal medicine is grounded in historical facts, it is far from folklore and there is clinical and scientific research to document its efficacy. This book outlines the many ways to use botanicals in healing in a practical and useful format. Herbs can be used as a tonic, as treatment, and as a preventative. The advantages of using an inexpensive, effective and less toxic substance are clearly beneficial.

'What is health and healing all about?', will become our major question for the 21st century. Protection of the rain forest, and fighting pollution, is vital if we are to prevent important healing plants from becoming extinct. Herbal medicine is thought to act by creating a homeostatic (metabolically balanced) healing process, rather than a suppressive one. By doing so, it promotes a balance towards health. Herbal medicine is therefore not anti-technology, but rather for self-care. We must integrate herbal therapies with conventional and complementary treatment. This holistic care gives us the knowledge and awareness to use appropriate botanical medicines. It also gives us the understanding of the relationship between ourselves, our environment and each other. Then as we heal ourselves, we can heal the planet.

**Edward J. Linkner M.D.**

*By protecting the natural world we live in, and taking care not to deplete the bounty it shares with us, we can begin to improve our own health and well-being.*

# INTRODUCTION

*The magic of plants has touched most of us. We marvel at their simple start as a seed,*

*the pattern of their unfolding leaves and the fragrance and delicacy of their flowers.*

*A field of wild flowers and grasses, or a forest of leafy trees, can uplift us.*

## WHAT IS HERBALISM?

Herbalism is the use of plants as medicines for healing. Its traditions are as old as mankind itself, and until the 18th century it was used as the most common form of medical treatment in Europe and North America. Today, in tribal cultures and among countries with Eastern traditions, such as China and India, medicinal herbs are still widely used. In more conventional medicine, pharmaceutical companies and doctors rely on plants for the basis of many drugs.

### EARLY HERBALISM

The first written herbal records date back well over 5000 years to the Sumerians, who described the use and actions of plants such as laurel, caraway and thyme. The ancient Egyptians used garlic, coriander, mint, castor oil and opium. In the Old Testament, too, there are references to the use of herbal medicines.

### ANCIENT CHINESE HERBALS

From manuscripts found in *Ma Wang Dui* Tomb Three in Hunan province, Chinese herbal medicine can be dated back to the 3rd century BC. These contained references to more than 250 medicinal substances and how to use them in prescriptions. The *Yellow Emperor's Inner Classic*, compiled over 2000 years ago, discusses the philosophical questions of health, illness, and the relationship of the human body to the cosmos. It also contains suggestions for using herbs, acupuncture, diet and exercise that are still relevant today. The traditional Chinese herbal has increased since then with the integration of substances from China's folk medicine and from other parts of Southeast Asia, India and the Middle East.

### GREEK AND ROMAN CONCEPTS

Ancient Greek and Roman medical practices are the basis for conventional medicine used in Western society today. Hippocrates, the Greek physician and 'father of medicine', advocated the use of a few simple herbal drugs, along with fresh air, rest and a healthy diet to aid the body in strengthening its own 'life force' to eliminate its problems. Galen, an influential Roman physician, believed in using larger doses of the remedies, including plant, animal, and mineral substances, as the means to heal diseases. The first European treatise on the properties and uses of medicinal herbs was *De Materia Medica*, written in the 1st century AD by the Greek physician Dioscorides. It was used well into the 17th century.

### THE MIDDLE AGES

The use of plants for medicines was common practice during the Middle Ages. The early Christian church discouraged this, preferring faith healing. However, the diligent work of the monks preserved many Greek medical manuscripts, and the monasteries, with their herb gardens, became local centres for herbal treatment. Folk medicine continued the use of herbal traditions, with the knowledge held by midwives and 'wise women'. Fear and superstition were rife, and many magical properties were attached to herbal medicine. Ultimately this led to the persecution and death of many women and healers. The use of herbs was passed on through apprenticeship and by word of mouth. So, during the Inquisition, when many herbalists were put to death, a great loss of herbal remedies occured.

## WESTERN HERBALISM

Despite the move in the 19th century toward the use of sophisticated drugs, 80 per cent of the world's population depends on medicines derived from traditional plant remedies. The recognition of the importance of ancient herbal traditions is increasing as people seek to find a greater understanding of themselves and their connection with the world around them.

## THE BALANCING NATURE OF HERBS

Plants take up substances from the earth and convert them into the vitamins, minerals, carbohydrates, proteins and fats which our bodies use for nourishment and healing. By using the whole plant or herb, we take in all the vital ingredients it carries. Most herbs contain several active substances, one of which usually dominates and determines its choice as a remedy. Other healing aspects of the herb should not be overlooked because they help the body to assimilate its benefits and buffer any side-effects.

## HERB COMBINATIONS

Herbs work synergistically, so combining them enhances each herb's properties, increasing its power to heal the body. For example, a good mixture to help induce sleep combines passiflora, valerian and hops. All three herbs have relaxant properties, but passiflora specializes in aiding sleep, valerian relaxes muscle tension, and hops have a marked effect on relaxing the nervous system.

## CHINESE HERBALISM

Chinese herbs are rarely used on their own; more commonly they are used in combination to form a Chinese prescription. The use of many herbs helps to achieve a balance within the prescription, and ensures that it enters the part of the body that needs healing. Herbs are described in terms of temperature, taste, what they do in the body and whether they affect the *yin*, *yang*, *qi* or blood.

## YIN AND YANG

The concept of *yin* and *yang* is embodied in Chinese philosophy. It maintains that all systems of the universe consist of two conflicting yet interdependent energies from which all forms of creation came. The nature of *yang* is hot, bright, upward and active, embodying the more masculine energy. The *yin* holds the cool, moist, inward and nourishing qualities, which are the more feminine principles. Astragalus is a *yang* herb used to warm, strengthen and raise the *qi*, or energy. Lycium fruit is a *yin* herb, whose actions work to restore depleted functions and to prevent further deterioration.

## QI AND BLOOD

In terms of Chinese medicine, *qi* is an energy which simultaneously manifests itself on the physical,

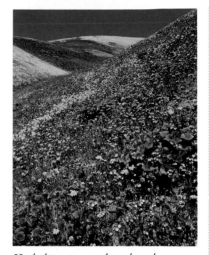

*Herbal treatments have been known and used for many centuries.*

emotional and spiritual levels, and is in a constant state of change. It is the vital force of existence. Blood is regarded as a denser, more material form of *qi*. *Qi* generates, moves and holds blood, yet blood nourishes *qi*, or, as the Chinese saying goes, 'Blood is the mother of *qi*.' Ginseng (*ren shen*) tones the *qi* of the body, including that of the lungs, digestion, and heart. Chinese angelica (*dang gui*) tones and moves the blood (it actually strengthens the *qi* of the blood).

## COMBINING WESTERN AND CHINESE HERBALISM

In this book, remedies include both Chinese and Western herbal suggestions. They can safely be used together as long as you have regard for any cautions and contra-indications, and use safe dosages. Many Chinese remedies are given as patent remedies, and in their pill form can be used easily and safely over a period of time. Western herbal teas can be drunk at the same time to help treat any ailment. Herbal tinctures are another easy way of combining Chinese and Western herbs.

# THINKING HOLISTICALLY

*By recognizing that there is a link between our mind and body, and to the world around us, we start to understand the importance of holistic health. By healing ourselves through working closely with gifts from nature, we learn to care for the environment.*

## HERBS AND THE ENVIRONMENT

Ecological awareness is necessary to avert a crisis on the planet on which we depend for life. Increasing pollution, the destruction of the rainforests, and the greenhouse effect could all have a potentially disastrous effect. Some herbs, which are more commonly regarded as weeds, are remarkably resilient. Any gardener knows that nettles, dock and couchgrass proliferate in most conditions. However, the more obscure healing plants are being lost as their environment is destroyed. Nature's gifts for the healing of more serious conditions, such as cancer and AIDS, are disappearing as we wipe out traditional tribal societies, losing their knowledge, lands and the plants they grow.

### LIVING IN HARMONY WITH NATURE

We need to find a way of living in harmony with the world around us to ensure a good quality of life. Plants provide us with oxygen through photosynthesis, as well as food and drink, shelter, coal, wood for fuel and medicines. From us they receive carbon dioxide, help with pollination and bacteria to break down dead remains and return their substances into the soil, which is the place of new life. As we strengthen our life force through connection with the plants and the world around us, we become more aware of our own vitality (or lack of it) and can find healing for ourselves.

### THE LIFE FORCE

The concept of the force of life is central to the philosophy of holistic healing. It is the essence that helps the body to heal itself. It is known in Chinese medicine as *qi*, and in Indian medicine as the vital energy, or *prana*. In a holistic approach, illness occurs when there is a disturbance within this life force. Symptoms of an illness help us to identify what we need in our lives to recover and restore our own healing energy.

### THE BODY IN HEALTH

Many of us may find it difficult to remember a time when we felt alive and vital. Childhood, or a long holiday, may have included moments when we felt a strong spark of life. Everyday life puts its demands on us, and we cope with them, putting aside the minor complaints of our bodies. It is when these complaints stop us from doing what we want to do that we seek help. By living in an unpolluted environment, eating a healthy diet, getting physical exercise, finding peace of mind and a positive attitude, we can do a great deal to restore good health. Herbal medicine offers much, helping us to take responsibility for our own health and offering simple treatments. Today, in North America, increasing numbers of Holistic Physicians combine conventional and alternative therapies in the prevention and treatment of diseases.

### ENVIRONMENTAL FACTORS

A pollution-free environment is hard to find these days, and it is not a possibility for everyone. So it is important to know the effect of pollution on our bodies. Some people, such as asthmatics, are obviously more sensitive, and they need to take extra care when pollution levels are high. Herbal treatments may help to boost immunity and calm reactions to environmental factors, but a long-term environmental solution is also needed.

### DIET

Food is an essential part of life, and a good diet goes a long way to preventing serious illness. A wholefood diet, preferably of organic foods, will help support good health. Fresh fruit and vegetables are necessary to supply essential vitamins and minerals and the roughage needed to clear wastes from the body. Avoid eating excessive amounts of foods high in refined sugars and flours, such as cakes, biscuits and sweets, as well as taking coffee, tea, alcohol and tobacco.

### EXERCISE

Our society has become more technological; the physical exercise that was once part of everyday life has been replaced by modern conveniences. Exercise has become an optional form of recreation, but we must nevertheless make a point of exercising because it helps us to relax and release tension, build up muscle tone, and strengthen our heart and lungs. It encourages the circulation of the blood and lymph systems so that all parts of our body become warm and our immunity is enhanced.

### PEACE OF MIND

Our physical, emotional and mental health are strongly connected. Many physical ailments, such as headaches, digestive complaints and low immunity, are linked to stress. Many herbal teas, baths and oils are mentioned in this book that help us to relax and to relieve tensions. It may also be important to talk through difficult situations, and counselling can help. Relaxation through yoga, meditation, and *t'ai chi* can be beneficial in restoring peace of mind; so can simple pleasures such as gardening, singing and walking.

### SPIRITUALITY

Belief in the greater good that is within all of us contributes to our spirituality. Although it can be difficult to hold on to this belief, the other option leaves us open to negativity, pessimism and cynicism. A positive state of mind, which carries with it hope, openness to different ways of living, and compassion for others and ourselves, encourages good feelings about life.

### DECIDING ON A HERBAL TREATMENT

There are many different ways of using herbs to provide a wide variety of treatments. Herbs can be taken as teas, wines and syrups, or used externally as baths, creams and lotions. The simplest and most common way of using herbs is as a herbal tea, and because of their increasing popularity, several of the

*Exercise strengthens the cardiovascular system and provides a good release for everyday stress and tension.*

*Symptoms caused by emotional difficulties may not respond to herbal treatments. Resolving your problems with a therapist or counsellor should enable you to respond more freely to the treatments.*

*A positive mental attitude, an openness to different ways of being, and compassion for others and ourselves, help to encourage good feelings about life.*

*Adopting a healthier lifestyle and learning to relax are essential parts of holistic treatment.*

*Good health lies in our own hands. Herbal remedies can help us to treat minor ailments before they develop into more serious problems.*

more widely known herb teas, such as peppermint, camomile and rosehip, can be bought in supermarkets. If you do not enjoy their taste, try peppermint or camomile as an essential oil in your bath.

### HERBS FOR PREVENTION

Taking herbs is an effective way to prevent illness and ailments. Garlic and echinacea both help to boost the immune system, and are especially helpful if there is a tendency to colds or infections during the winter. If you are prone to anxiety, and know that you are facing a particularly difficult time, try drinking camomile tea to help you relax. Use lavender oil in a bath or on your pillow to help you

sleep at night so that you get a good night's rest and can cope better. Herbs can be used at the first sign of a complaint to avoid a more serious illness. Drink hot peppermint tea with honey and a few slices of ginger root at the first sniffle of a cold, or a hot tea of boneset to ward off flu symptoms.

### USING HERBS SAFELY

Herbal medicine, like any other medicine, deserves care and respect. The Herbal Directory (*see* pp.100–151) lists the herbs most frequently suggested in this book, and details any cautions or contra-indications about taking it. Take the time to look at these when you have decided on the herbs best suited for your treatment. The

dosages are also given for each herb and must be closely followed. Standard dosages for infusions, decoctions, tinctures, wines, baths, inhalations and Chinese patent remedies are given in the Herbal Methods section (*see* p.16). Remember that dosages will vary with age, so children and the elderly should take less than an adult. If a woman is breastfeeding, any herb she takes will be excreted in her milk. It is, therefore, important to seek professional advice. If you are taking homeopathic remedies, you should consult a homeopath or herbal practitioner before beginning any herbal treatment. If you are in any doubt about using a herb, consult a professional herbalist.

# HOW TO USE THIS BOOK

❦

*This book is divided into three main sections. You may choose to read parts of it for general interest, or consult it for treatment for different ailments. It is a reference for herbs that may be used simply and effectively to treat a wide variety of complaints. It seeks to give you a greater understanding of how the body works and how to use herbal medicine.*

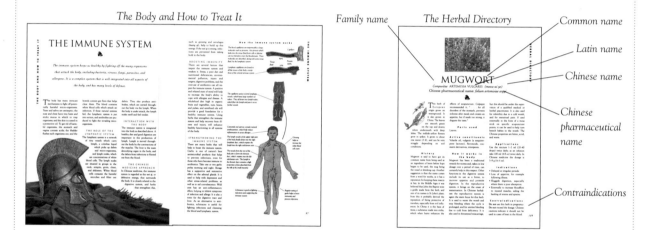

*The Body and How to Treat It*

Family name    *The Herbal Directory*    Common name

Latin name

Chinese name

Chinese pharmaceutical name

Contraindications

### HERBAL METHODS

This section describes different techniques for preparing herbs, from the making of infusions, or herbal teas, to the more complicated processes of preparing ointments and creams. It gives useful recipes, such as an iron tonic medicinal wine that uses nettle, and an eyewash for tired eyes that contains camomile. Dosages, which differ for the various preparations and with the age of the patient, are also given, and these must be consulted before using any herbal treatment.

### THE BODY AND HOW TO TREAT IT

This section discusses different systems in the body, looking at how they work and suggesting the herbal remedies that can help with the ailments related to them. Suggestions for preventing illness and keeping the body healthy, as well as advice regarding diet and lifestyle, are also given. Before taking any herbal treatment, check the herbs recommended in the Herbal Directory (pp.100–151) to ensure that you take the correct dosage and that there are no contraindications.

### HERBAL DIRECTORY

This section gives specific information on the herbs recommended in this book, including a brief description of the herb, its use, how to apply it, any contraindications and appropriate dosages. Herbs used or mentioned in the book but not included in the Directory are described briefly in the Additional Herbs list (p.152). The Glossary (p.156) explains commonly used herbal terminology. This section also includes instructions on how to make remedies from items found in most kitchens, and suggestions for herbal first-aid treatments.

# HERBAL METHODS

## WHERE TO GET HERBS

There are several ways of obtaining herbs. The first is to pick them from the wild, following the guidelines below. This will enable you to have the benefit of fresh herbs, which can also be stored and dried. Second, you can buy dried herbs from a shop or by mail order. Third, you may decide to grow your own herbs. This will give you the advantage of using fresh herbs grown on your doorstep, enabling you to enjoy their foliage and scents, as well as reaping the medicinal benefits.

### PICKING YOUR OWN HERBS

A few common-sense rules about picking herbs will ensure that you are not depleting the countryside and that nature's gifts are preserved for everyone's pleasure and benefit.

- It is important never to strip an area of its natural resources.
- Do not uproot plants and take them home with you; it is better to select a few specimens for harvesting and to leave the rest to multiply.
- Harvest only common, plentiful plants – the weeds of the countryside – not rare or scarce plants. Be sure to check local regulations on gathering herbs.
- Always ensure that the plant you are harvesting is the plant you require – double-check, using a good field guide to wild plants.
- Better still, go on a herb walk with an experienced herbalist, who will identify plants for you.
- Above all, make sure you are not harvesting a protected species.

### CHOOSING HEALTHY HERBS

Check that no pesticides or herbicides have been used in the area, and that the plants are not growing close to industrial buildings or busy roads, which may emit waste products or pollution. Try to ensure that the herbs are free from animal droppings or insect damage, and are generally healthy, fresh-looking plants.

### THE GROWING LIFE OF THE HERB

It is useful to familiarize yourself with the growing life of the plant you are thinking of using. Knowing the plant's habitat and growing season will add greatly to your knowledge of its medicinal value and benefits. Gather the herbs after the first dew has evaporated, but before the sun is fully on them. This will ensure that they are dry, and that they will not have lost any of their precious constituents.

### WHICH PART OF THE PLANT TO USE

It is important to find out which part of the

plant is best suited for your purpose. For example, while the dandelion leaf acts as a diuretic and would be useful for those suffering from high blood pressure, the root is suitable for treating the liver and acts as a mild laxative.

## SEASONAL CHANGES

Decide which parts of the plants you intend to use, and check the time of year most suitable for harvesting them. For instance, roots are better harvested in the autumn, when the aerial part of the plant has died, leaving the goodness in the roots, to be stored until spring. The leaves of a plant are best harvested in the spring. Flowers, on the other hand, are at their best later in the season. Berries should be picked when they are ripe. Bark should be purchased commercially, since cutting a tree may damage or kill it.

## BUYING HERBS

You may be able to purchase dried herbs locally or from a mail order company. Either is likely to be a good source, but be sure to compare the quality by looking at, smelling, and tasting the herbs to ensure value for money. Dried herbs do not have a shelf-life of longer than about a year, so look for colour: the flowers should retain some of their colour and the leaves should still have some green in them; if a marigold looks pale and insipid instead of a glorious orange, it may have been stored for too long. The herbs also should still have a scent. Lastly, test by taste: when infused or decocted you should be able to tell the herbs apart; they should not taste dull or lacking in flavor.

## DRYING HERBS

If you decide to use herbs fresh, you need to use them quite quickly or they will decay. Alternatively, you can dry the plant carefully in a warm cupboard or spread it on brown paper on a rack in a warm, shady place. When drying flower heads, such as marigold, or large leaves, set them out so they do not overlap and air can circulate around them. Leave them to dry for one to three weeks. If mould appears, it means there is too much moisture circulating and you will have to discard the batch and repeat the process. When drying a plant with small flowers, such as lavender, or leaves, it is best to dry them in bunches of four or five, hanging upside down by their stems in a paper bag. Ensure that the bag covers the flower heads or leaves, then secure it with an elastic band. Roots should be cleaned and cut into small pieces, which you can dry on a baking tray in the oven at about 120°F (50°C) until they are brittle. If they remain soft, they still retain moisture, so check them at intervals. Be patient; too much heat too fast may destroy some of the plant's delicate constituents.

## STORING HERBS

When the herbs are dry, store them in a clean, dry jar, preferably of dark glass, and keep them out of the sunlight. When buying dried herbs from a supplier, transfer them into a clean, dry jar with a close-fitting lid. Store in a dry place, out of the sunlight. Never leave herbs in plastic containers or plastic wrapping, since this shortens their shelf-life. You can store herbs in paper bags, but you must take extra care to safeguard them from damp and insects. Label the container with the name of the herb and the date, or you may forget which herbs are which, and how long you have been storing them.

## GROWING HERBS

If you want to buy an already growing plant, check that the specimen is from a good supplier and is healthy and free from pests. Plants that have been grown organically will be free from pesticide or herbicide residues, and will not have been grown with chemical fertilizers. This will ensure that only the most natural and healthy substances enter your body.

*Children respond well to herbal remedies. Always check the correct dosage for each herb based on the age of your child.*

## DOSAGE

The dosage will depend on the method of preparation and the age of the person taking the herb. When following dosages and recipes, it is important to use just one system of measurement, so stick to either metric or imperial.

Infusions and decoctions are taken in cupfuls or millilitres. Each cupful is approximately 200 ml (8 fl oz) and a potful is approximately 600 ml (1¼ pints).

Tinctures are given in much smaller dosages, usually teaspoons or drops. One teaspoon is 5 ml and one millilitre is about 20 drops.

Medicinal wines are usually taken as one sherry glassful (approximately 70 ml) a day.

Syrups are taken by the teaspoonful. One to two teaspoons may be taken three times a day.

### Guidelines for dosages

| | |
|---|---|
| **Babies to six months** | Should have herbal remedies only under guidance of an experienced practitioner. |
| **Babies to one year** | One-tenth of adult dose. If the mother is breastfeeding, the infant will receive the correct amount if the mother takes the normal dosage. It is important to consult a qualified practitioner. |
| **Children one to six** | One-third the normal adult dose. |
| **Children six to twelve** | One-half the normal adult dose. |
| **Adults** | Infusions    3–4 cups* a day<br>Decoctions 2–3 cups a day<br>Tincture    5 ml (1 tsp) 2–3 times a day |
| **Over 70s** | Infusions    2–3 cups a day<br>Decoctions 1–2 cups a day<br>Tincture    5 ml (1 tsp) 2–3 times a day<br>*A cup is approximately 200 ml (8 fl oz) |
| **Pregnancy** | Many herbs are useful in pregnancy, but it is advisable to check all remedies with a qualified practitioner before use. |

# INFUSIONS

❧

*Infusions are used to prepare the delicate parts of a plant, such as the leaves, flowers and seeds, which break down easily to release their medicinal elements into the water. An infusion is also known as a tea or a tisane, a time-honoured method of preparing herbs.*

## MAKING AN INFUSION

If making the tisane in a pot, do not use one in which regular tea is made because the tannin residue will overpower the ingredients in the herbal tea. If you are making tea in a teacup, you will need to cover it with a lid or a saucer. This is because some of the constituents of the tea include volatile oils, which evaporate in steam, and so the tea will lose much of its medicinal value if left uncovered. The tea may be drunk hot or left to cool, then placed in the refrigerator and drunk during the day. It may be kept for up to 24 hours.

### Method

*When using a teapot, you will need about 600 ml (1¼ pints) of boiling water and approximately 20 g (1 oz) of dried, or 30 g (1½ oz) of fresh herbs.*

This will make enough tea for three or four cups a day. You may use a single herb or two or three in equal quantities, to make up the amount.

*If making an infusion in a cup, use approximately 2 g (1–2 tsp) of dried, or 3 g (2–3 tsp) of fresh, herbs per cup.*

Drink a cup of tea two or three times a day, depending on the appropriate dose (*see* p.16).

To prepare a pot of tea, first warm the pot, then place the herbs in it and add freshly boiled water. Replace the lid and leave the herbs to steep for 10 minutes. Using a tea-strainer, pour the tea into a cup, adding honey as a sweetener if required. To make a single cup, place the herbs in a tea-strainer on the cup and pour over freshly boiled water until it covers the herbs. Cover the cup and leave the tea for 10 minutes; add honey as a sweetener if desired.

### COLD AND FLU TEA

*One-half yarrow*
*One-half elderflower*
*Pinch of peppermint*
*This cold and flu remedy, suitable for adults, will lower a fever, reduce nasal catarrh and promote sweating to help cleanse and restore the system.*

*When selecting appropriate herbs for your infusion, choose one which has a pleasant taste, such as lemon balm, so that your tea will be refreshing as well as healthy.*

# DECOCTIONS

*A decoction is used to prepare the more resistant parts of a plant —*

*the bark, roots, rhizomes and berries — where the constituents in the*

*herb are more difficult to extract. Decoctions are always boiled for a*

*minimum of 10 minutes.*

*Decoctions are made in larger quantities and last longer than infusions because the boiling process sterilizes the liquid.*

### Method
*20 g (1 oz) of dried, or 40 g (2 oz) fresh herb to about 750 ml (1½ pints) of water*

Sections of root or bark should be chopped as finely as possible in order to allow the boiling water to extract the maximum from the plant. Place in a pan, cover with cold water and bring to the boil. Cover the pan with a tight-fitting lid and simmer for the required period. Allow the preparation to cool before straining, pressing out as much liquid from the residue as possible in order not to waste any of the valuable properties extracted.

If you wish to combine the properties of two herbs, for instance, a root and a flower or leaf, the flower or leaf should be added at the end of the simmering period. The mixture should then be left, covered, for 10 minutes. It is possible to keep this mixture for the same period as a normal decoction because the liquid has been sterilized.

### STRESS AND ANXIETY DRINK
*One-third valerian root decoction*
*One third skullcap infusion*
*One-third verbena infusion*
*This remedy for adults is helpful during times of stress. It will lessen anxiety, and provide a tonic for the nervous system.*

# TINCTURES

*Tinctures can be used to prepare roots or leaves. They include alcohol and water to extract properties from the herbs which would not be available if a water preparation alone was used. It is possible to replace the alcohol with glycerol or vinegar.*

## STORAGE AND DOSAGE

As a tincture will last for up to two years, it is a very convenient method of preparation if you intend long-term use of the herbs. A tincture is much stronger than either an infusion or a decoction, and is taken in millilitres (ml) or teaspoons (tsp) depending on the herb used. Use a dropper to measure amounts. In general, 20 drops = 1 ml. The average dose will vary between 1 ml (⅕ tsp) three times a day, and 5 ml (1 tsp) three times a day, but this will depend on the herb, so always check the individual herbal dosages (*see* Herbal Directory).

### Method

*200 g (8 oz) dried herb*
*250 ml (½ pint) alcohol\**
*750 ml (1½ pints) water*
*\*The alcohol should be at least 30 per cent proof in order to extract constituents and to preserve them. Suitable mediums include gin and vodka. Never use industrial alcohol.*

*The ratio of herb to liquid is one part herb to one part liquid. The liquid is made up of 25 per cent alcohol and 75 per cent water.*

Finely chop the herbs and place them in a glass vessel or jar with a tightly fitting lid. Cover the herbs with the liquid and secure the lid.

The jar should be placed in a warm, dark place for 14 days. Shake the mixture every two or three days. At the end of this time, strain the mixture into a clean jar, keeping the remains of the wet herbs to one side. These can be pressed to extract every drop of the tincture by using a wine press if you have one, or by wrapping the herbs in a muslin cloth and wringing out the last few drops. Keep the tincture in a coloured glass jar or bottle, and store in a dark place.

## TINCTURE FOR SLEEPLESSNESS

*100 g (4 oz) German camomile*
*250 ml (½ pint) vodka*
*750 ml (1½ pints) water*
*This tincture is excellent as an aid to restful sleep. Begin by taking 5 ml (1 tsp) approximately 20 minutes before going to bed. If this is not effective take a further 5 ml (1 tsp). You may take a maximum of 15 ml (3 tsp) in one night. The next evening you could begin with 10 ml (2 tsp) and so on until you find the most effective dose for your needs.*

*Always label tinctures with the name of the herb and the date prepared. A notebook is useful to record ailments treated and successful herbal combinations.*

# MEDICINAL WINES

*Wines have long been used for medicinal purposes. There are two*

*main ways to make a medicinal wine. The first is to use a*

*commercially bought wine — preferably organic — and steep herbs*

*in it. The second is to make the wine yourself.*

### Method 1
*100 g (4 oz) dried herbs*
*1 litre (2 pints) red or white wine*

Place the herbs in a glass jar with a tight-fitting lid and cover with the wine. Once sealed, the jar should be left for at least two weeks to steep. The liquid should then be filtered and the liquid rebottled and stored for use as required.

### Method 2
*1 whole root ginger, peeled*
*1 kg (2¼ lb) sugar*
*rind and juice of 2 lemons and*
*2 oranges*
*1 banana*
*good pinch cayenne*
*pepper*
*200 g (8 oz) raisins*
*or golden raisins*
*yeast compound*
*1 large pot of tea*

First squeeze the oranges and lemons, then slice the banana. Grate the ginger. Chop the skins of the lemons and oranges, and add the raisins, cayenne pepper and 450g (1 lb) of sugar. Place in a demijohn. Make a large pot of regular tea and pour over the ingredients in the demijohn. Allow the sugar to dissolve and the mixture to cool slightly, then add a general-purpose yeast compound. Loosely stopper the demijohn. Leave to ferment for at least a week, adding tea until the demijohn is about two-thirds full. Then strain out the fruit and ginger and replace the liquid. Add the rest of the sugar and top up with tea if necessary. Continue to ferment for

another week, then bottle. This wine combines the qualities of ginger and cayenne. Ginger is a warming, circulatory stimulant. It is excellent for colds, since it is anti-inflammatory, antiseptic and helps to stop coughing. Cayenne is recommended for sore throats and as a remedy for poor circulation.

### CHESTY COUGH REMEDY (METHOD 1)
*100 g (4 oz) dried elecampane root (or*
*200 g (8 oz) fresh elecampane root)*
*1 litre (2 pints) white wine*
*This tonic wine is useful for a persistent*
*chesty cough, since it both soothes*
*inflamed tissue and is an expectorant.*

### IRON TONIC RECIPE (METHOD 1)
*50 g (approx. 2 oz) dried nettles*
*50 g (approx. 2 oz) chopped apricots*
*1 litre (2 pints) red wine*
*This wine can be used as a tonic for*
*anemic conditions where there is*
*lethargy and tiredness, and also for*
*dry eczema.*

*Red wines are believed to have a beneficial effect on the heart, while white grapes are thought to be good for the immune system, 'mopping up' harmful toxins.*

# GARGLES AND MOUTHWASHES

*A gargle or mouthwash can be made from an infusion, a decoction or a diluted tincture. It may be used for a variety of complaints associated with the mouth and throat. A gargle may help to soothe a sore and irritated throat associated with a cold or laryngitis.*

*A mouthwash or gargle made from an infusion, decoction or diluted tincture can be used to keep breath fresh and to relieve tender gums or troublesome mouth ulcers.*

need further treatment, for example, for a depleted immune system.

### Methods

#### INFUSIONS/ DECOCTIONS

Make an infusion of herb tea, allow it to stand for 10 minutes, then leave it to cool as required. Strain, and use as a gargle or mouthwash.

#### TINCTURES

*Dilute 5 ml (1 tsp) of the chosen tincture in 100 ml (4 fl oz) of water, and use as indicated.*

#### MOUTH ULCER RECIPE

*2 ml (½ tsp) sage tincture*
*2 ml (½ tsp) marigold tincture*
*1 ml (⅕ tsp) myrrh tincture*
*100 ml (4 fl oz) water*
*This preparation can be used either as a mouthwash, when diluted, or neat as a lotion to dab directly on the ulcers using a piece of cottonwool. It combines antiseptic and wound-healing properties and is an excellent remedy for mouth ulcers. When used neat, the tincture may sting slightly.*

#### MOUTH-FRESHENING RECIPE

*1 cup sage tea*
*A simple infusion of sage is ideal to relieve a sore throat or simply to refresh the mouth. The volatile oils in sage help to cleanse and protect against bacteria, which can cause infection and damage teeth or gums.*

### ANTISEPTIC PROPERTIES

Choose herbs that are known for their antiseptic properties. It is safe to swallow some of the liquid as you are gargling, bearing in mind the daily recommended dosage of the herb used and any general cautions (*see* Herbal Directory). A gargle may be used four or five times a day. Where there is persistent gum trouble, seek further help from your dentist or doctor to rule out any underlying problems. If mouth ulcers continually recur, this can suggest a problem which may

# EYEWASHES

*An eyewash or bath is a refreshing way to relieve tired eyes*

*caused by working under artificial lights and at computer screens.*

*An eyewash can also relieve irritation caused by*

*pollen or pollution.*

### HYGIENE

To ensure that no bacteria come into contact with the eyes, all utensils, such as eyebaths, must be sterilized by boiling for 10 minutes before use. If you have only one eyebath, treat one eye, then re-sterilize the eyebath before bathing the other eye so that infection is not passed on.

### PREPARING AN EYEWASH

The eyewash is prepared in the same way as an infusion, but first boil the water for 10 minutes before pouring it over the herbs to be sure the water is sterilized. The liquid needs to be strained very carefully to avoid particles from the herbs being transferred to the eyes. Allow the liquid to cool before applying. If using eyewashes frequently, add a little salt to the wash to help re-balance the eye's natural fluid.

### USING THE EYEBATH

Place the liquid in the eyebath and cover the eye, tipping the head back to allow the solution to bathe the eye gently. If any discomfort or irritation occurs when using an eyewash stop treatment immediately. If an infected condition persists, seek advice from a qualified practitioner.

### Method 1

*Make a compress by soaking a piece of cotton or lint in the eyewash infusion. Allow to cool, and place on the eyelids for 10–15 minutes.*

### Method 2

*Prepare an infusion as described. Leave to cool until lukewarm, then fill an eyebath and bathe eyes. Twice a day should be sufficient.*

### TIRED EYES REMEDY (METHOD 1)

*1 cup camomile tea*

*This is a refreshing way to ease sore or tired eyes after a hard day at work, especially after looking at a computer screen. Camomile has anti-inflammatory properties to soothe and revitalize your eyes.*

### CONJUNCTIVITIS REMEDY (METHOD 2)

*½ cup eyebright tea*
*½ cup marigold tea*

*This remedy combines eyebright to reduce inflammation and marigold for its antiseptic, healing qualities.*

*Care for your eyes by taking time out to relieve stress and tension. Use an eyebath or compress to relax and restore vitality to your eyes.*

# BATHS

*Baths can be cleansing, relaxing or revitalizing. When you add*

*herbs to your bath, you can enhance the benefits of your usual*

*bathtime routine. Either infusions or decoctions can be used in baths*

*or you may wish to try the benefits of essential oils.*

*If a whole-body bath is not possible,
for example, in cases of illness or
infirmity, a hand or foot bath can
provide relief.*

### WHOLE-BODY BATH

To your normal bath water add the equivalent of one potful, about 600 ml (1¼ pints), herbal infusion which has been strained. Mix well. Alternatively, add roughly five drops essential oils to the bath while the water is running. (Do not use essential oils in baby baths as a baby can ingest the oils through mouth/hand contact.) This eases aching muscles and limbs. You should not allow the bath to become too cold or the benefits will be lost. Try an infusion of lavender to relax in the evening, rosemary to invigorate in the morning, and thyme to soothe aching muscles.

### HAND BATH

Using a suitable bowl or basin, immerse the entire hand up to the wrist in the cooled, strained herbal infusion. Make sure your position is comfortable. Do not sit with your hand and wrist at an awkward angle, but allow it to rest in a relaxed manner. For hot, painful arthritic joints, a cooling infusion such as peppermint is indicated, while for a cold, aching joint, a hotter infusion of ginger is warming. At all times, however, you should feel relaxed. The immersion should last between 5 and 10 minutes. Make sure you dry your hands thoroughly after the bath.

### FOOT BATH

This is especially good for relaxing tired, aching feet at the end of a long day. Treating your feet will enable the rest of your body to feel the benefits as well. One of the simplest remedies for a cold is to sit with your feet in a bowl of fairly hot water to which a heaped teaspoon of mustard powder has been added. Sit for 10 minutes, then dry and wrap the feet warmly.

### BODY WASH

Prepare an infusion of your chosen herb, strain, and, with a clean cloth, gently bathe the selected area. Tepid water is best for this type of wash. Dry gently.

# INHALATIONS

*A steam inhalation can be used to relieve conditions such as colds and flu, catarrh, sinusitus and many other problems. The steam helps to relax the airways and benefits mucous membranes.*

## Method

Approximately two potfuls – 1 litre (2 pints) – of liquid are needed. Prepare the infusion by adding the freshly boiled water to the herb, then pouring it immediately into a suitable bowl placed ready for use. (It is best to take the infusion to the bowl rather than carrying a heavy, rather hot, bowl from room to room.) If using essential oils, first boil the water and pour into the bowl, then add between three to six drops of the oil to the liquid and stir. Sit comfortably and place a large towel or cloth over your head and the bowl so that none of the steam can escape. Continue this treatment for about 10 minutes or until the water cools, but do come up for air if you need to. Afterwards, sit in a warmed room for about half an hour to allow your respiratory system to adjust to the ambient temperature.

## CONGESTION RECIPE

*2 drops thyme essential oil*
*2 drops eucalyptus essential oil*
*1 litre (2 pints) water*
*The properties of thyme make it an excellent decongestant for a stuffy or blocked nose or sinuses, for example, in allergic conditions. Eucalyptus oil contains ingredients which help to relax tight airways and aid breathing, as well as having antiseptic properties that are particularly good for flus and colds.*

## VAPORIZERS/ DIFFUSERS

An oil vaporizer/diffuser placed in a room is ideal if you wish to use a less-concentrated inhalation. Vaporizers are easy to find, and come in many different designs and shapes. Generally, they consist of a small nightlight candle with a bowl above, into which the water and essential oil are poured. It is important to fill the bowl. A half-filled bowl may crack because the light will continue to burn after the water has evaporated. Use between 1 and 6 drops of essential oil. If a vaporizer is not available, a bowl filled with boiling water to which the essential oil is added will allow the vapour to diffuse throughout the room. A drop or two of oil on a piece of cottonwool or clean cloth placed above (not on) a radiator will have much the same effect.

## TENSION RECIPE

*3–5 drops lavender essential oil*
*Bowl of hot water/diffuser*
*Lavender has a calming, sedative effect. If tension prevents you from winding down after a hard day, add it to a bowl of water or a diffuser, and allow your cares to drift away.*

## HERBAL HEALING

The addition of a herbal remedy to a steam inhalation helps to ease congestion, clear mucus, and relieve respiratory stress. Younger children with colds may benefit from being taken into a steamy bathroom to ease breathing and other symptoms.

*Lavender has a calming, sedative effect. Use it as an essential oil in a steam inhalation to relieve a headache caused by stress and to aid restful sleep.*

# INFUSED OILS

🎵

*Infused oils are altogether different from essential oils and can be made easily and cheaply at home. They can be used for massage or as a base oil to which essential oils can be added.*

*Hot and cold oil infusions can be used for massage and also as a base when making creams and ointments.*

### WHICH OILS TO USE
The best oils for infusions are vegetable, for example, sunflower or soya. Use olive oil only for cold infusions. Oils last for about a year.

### CAUTION
Handle hot oils carefully. *Never* use infused oils internally or allow them to come into contact with delicate membranes, such as the eyes.

### COLD AND HOT OILS
There are two ways of making an infused oil: a cold preparation in which the oils are heated by the sun, and a hot preparation in which the oils are heated gently on the stove.

**Method**
#### COLD OILS
This method is very easy but slow. Take a clean, dry jar with a tight-fitting lid and pack it full with your chosen herb. Gently pour the oil into the jar, covering the herb fully. Put the lid on and place it on a warm, sunny windowsill for about two weeks, shaking and turning the jar daily. At the end of this time you will need to strain the oil carefully, using a muslin bag or cloth stretched over a bowl. Make sure all the plant material is removed, and squeeze out every last drop of oil to get the maximum benefit. Store the oil in a dark bottle away from sunlight. Do not forget to label and date your preparation.

### HOT OILS
*100 g (4 oz) dried herb*
*or 200 g (8 oz) fresh herb*
*400 ml (16 fl oz) vegetable oil*

This process is somewhat more complicated but gives a good-quality oil. The method uses a double boiler – a pan filled with water, brought to a boil then allowed to simmer gently, over which a larger pan or glass bowl is placed. The vegetable oil and herb are put into this, so the oil never comes into direct contact with the heat. The pan or bowl containing the oil and herb should be covered with a tight-fitting lid. The mixture is then left for a minimum of two hours, and allowed to cool before the oil is filtered into a clean bowl, using a cloth or straining bag. The used herb should be discarded and the process repeated, using fresh herbs, to produce a double-strength oil. Again, the oil should be filtered and the used herb thrown away. Bottle the oil in a dark glass jar, and store out of the sunlight.

### NERVE TONIC OIL
*St John's wort flowers*
*Vegetable oil*
*The flowers of St. John's wort are yellow, but as the plant oils are diffused into the vegetable oil, the colour will become deep red. This oil is excellent for gently massaging into areas where there is nerve strain or pain, for example, in cases of repetitive strain injury or neuralgia.*

# OINTMENTS

*Ointments are oil-based preparations which, in addition to aiding*

*the healing process, form a protective layer on the skin. This makes*

*them ideally suited for use where areas of skin are exposed to the*

*elements, for chapped lips, for example, or dry eczema.*

### PATCH TEST FOR SENSITIVE SKIN

Homemade herbal creams and ointments are ideal for those with sensitive or allergic skin because you can choose your own ingredients and minimize the use of additives or preservatives, which can cause irritation. However, before using any remedy on the skin first try a patch test. Apply a little of the ointment or cream to an area of skin and leave it for 24 hours. If any reaction occurs, discontinue its use. Seek medical advice if the irritation persists.

### Method

*200 ml (8 fl oz) infused oil*
*25 g (1 oz) beeswax*
*2–5 drops essential oil*

Fill a pan with water, bring it to a boil and then reduce it to a simmer. Place another pan or glass bowl over the boiling water and pour in the oil. Grate the beeswax and add it gradually, stirring until the wax is melted. Add any essential oils you wish to use. Remove the bowl from the heat, and, while still warm, carefully pour the contents into a clean glass jar and allow to set. Seal the jar, then label and date it.

*Homemade ointments and creams provide a gentle alternative to commercially made products. They can bring relief to skin that has been affected by sun, age, food and soap.*

### OINTMENT FOR CUTS AND SCRAPES

*200 ml (8 fl oz) infused marigold oil*
*25 g (1 oz) beeswax*
*2 drops lavender essential oil*
*This ointment combines the anti-bacterial healing properties of marigold with the astringent and anti-inflammatory qualities of lavender.*

# CREAMS

*Skin creams are preparations which combine oil and a water-based medium to create a mixture which nourishes and enriches the skin. Creams that are firm act as a barrier against the elements, while those of liquid consistency can be used to cleanse and moisturize.*

### PREPARING A CREAM

Creams are slightly more difficult to prepare than ointments since the oil and water base must be carefully blended or the two ingredients will separate out. The water base portion of the recipe could be either an infusion or a decoction of the chosen herbs. An agent is required to facilitate the blending process, usually emulsifying wax.

### HOW MUCH TO MAKE

Because a cream includes water, its shelf-life will be less than that of an ointment; it is better, therefore, to prepare only a small quantity. To help preserve and enhance the quality of the cream it is possible to add an essential oil. A cream should always be stored in a cool place or in the refrigerator.

### Method

*7 parts infusion/decoction*
*2 parts oil*
*1 part emulsifying wax*

This ratio is always the same whatever amounts you are using. If you are using teaspoons, the recipe will use seven teaspoons of infusion, two teaspoons of oil, and one teaspoon of emulsifying wax. Mix in three drops of essential oil to each 30 g (1¼ oz) made. Fill a pan with water, bring to a boil, and simmer.

Place a second pan or bowl over the first and pour in the oil and infusion. Gradually add in the emulsifying wax, stirring until it is dissolved. Remove the bowl from the heat and place it in a bowl filled with cold water. It is important to keep stirring the mixture or the ingredients will separate out; as it cools, the cream will gradually take on a thicker consistency. Add the essential oil and mix well. Spoon the mixture into glass jars, replace the lids, label and date. Store in the refrigerator or other cool place.

### SOOTHING CREAM

*7 teaspoons chickweed infusion*
*2 teaspoons oil*
*1 teaspoon emulsifying wax*
*3 drops camomile essential oil*
*Chickweed is extremely cooling and is noted for its effective relief of itching. Camomile essential oil combines anti-allergenic and anti-inflammatory properties with the preservation and enhancement of the fragrance of the cream.*

*Creams are particularly good for soothing an area of skin that is irritated or dry. A patch test should always be done first.*

# SYRUPS

*Syrups are soothing mixtures which are popular with adults and children alike. You can turn an infusion, a decoction or a tincture into a syrup by combining the liquid-based remedy with sugar or honey. This will also improve the taste of less-pleasant herbs.*

**Method**
INFUSION-BASED
SYRUP
*200 ml (8 fl oz) infusion
200 g (8 oz) sugar/honey*

For this type of syrup, you will need equal amounts of infusion and sugar. Prepare your infusion in the usual manner, but leave it to steep for 15 rather than 10 minutes.

*Syrups are sweet and easily swallowed, so they are useful in relieving coughs and sore throats, particularly when treating children.*

Strain the tea as usual, taking care to press out as much of the liquid as possible. The liquid should then be heated gently in a pan and the sugar or honey added. Stir constantly to dissolve all the sugar, taking care not to boil the mixture. Allow the syrup to cool, then pour it into bottles, seal and label them. Store in a cool, dark place. (Take care when sealing the bottle that the lid is left slightly loose, since tightly stoppered bottles have been known to explode.)

**Method**
DECOCTION-BASED
SYRUP
This method is exactly the same as for infusion-based syrups except that the decoction should be simmered for 30 minutes.

**Method**
TINCTURE-BASED
SYRUP
*100 ml (4 fl oz) water
200 g (8 oz) sugar/honey
100 ml (4 fl oz) tincture*

First prepare the syrup and then add the tincture. Boil the water, and add it to the sugar or honey, which has been placed in another pan. Stir until all the sugar is dissolved, and remove the pan from the heat. Allow it to cool, then stir in the tincture. Bottle, seal and label as before. The quantities are always used in the same ratio: that is, one part tincture to three parts syrup.

RECIPE FOR COUGH
SYRUP (INFUSION)
*200 ml (8 fl oz) infusion of thyme
200 g (8 oz) unrefined sugar
This remedy uses the antiseptic and expectorant qualities of thyme to relieve coughs and sore throats and is especially good for children.*

# VINEGARS

*Vinegars can be used in a similar way to tinctures and can provide an alternative for those who do find neither the alcoholic nor glycerine preparations suitable. Vinegar contains acetic acid, which helps to preserve and extract the essential ingredients of herbs.*

### PREPARATION

Use a jar or bottle with a wide mouth. Choose your herb, making sure it is as dry as possible. Place the herb in the jar and top up with the vinegar. Store for a minimum of two weeks (some sources recommend one or two months) in a dark place, shaking every day. Then strain off the liquid and bottle it. The vinegar should be left for a further two weeks before using.

### DOSAGE

Herb vinegars can be taken internally in the same way as tinctures, that is, by the teaspoonful, added to salads and soups, or as an ingredient in pickles. Externally they can be added to bathwater, and used as a lotion or even a hair rinse. The recipes given below show how versatile vinegars can be.

### ITCHY-SKIN LOTION

*Elderflower blossoms*
*Cider vinegar*
*The flowers of the elder tree are noted for their anti-inflammatory action. Especially valued for internal use in allergic conditions, the flowers can also be used in a vinegar-base as an external wash to calm and soothe itching skin, especially in cases of allergic reactions.*
*It is useful to have some on hand as a first-aid measure, to alleviate the painful burning of insect stings.*

### DRY-SCALP RINSE

*Nettle tops*
*White wine vinegar*
*The astringent properties of nettle and the softening effects of vinegar combine to help bring a shine to dull hair and to encourage circulation in a dry scalp. Add a little of the vinegar to your final rinsing water.*

### SALAD DRESSING

*2 cloves garlic, peeled and chopped*
*200 ml (8 fl oz) white wine vinegar*
*Garlic is noted for its healing properties, but its pungent odour can be problematic. Including it in a vinegar dressing and adding it to salads often proves a more palatable way of taking it. Medicinal benefits include an antibiotic effect and an anticholesterol action. It is also a good remedy for chest and other respiratory infections.*

*In addition to their medicinal function, vinegars are an interesting way to complement foods. Apple cider or wine vinegars, preferably organic, are most versatile.*

# POULTICES AND COMPRESSES

*Traditionally, poultices are used to draw out toxins from the body, promote circulation and aid healing. Poultices and compresses are applied in the same way, but are prepared differently and perform different functions.*

RECIPE FOR
DRAWING PASTE
*Equal parts of:*
*Marshmallow root powder*
*Slippery elm powder*
*Water*
*This recipe combines the drawing qualities of marshmallow with the demulcent, soothing properties of slippery elm. Use it for drawing out splinters, insect stings and boils. It can also be used to counter irritation from insect bites.*

## COMPRESSES

Compresses are also applied directly to the skin, but in this instance it is the liquid from the mixture, rather than the herb, which is used. Again, a compress can utilize either an infusion, a decoction, or a tincture. If using a tincture, it should be diluted with a little water. Once the liquid is prepared, a clean cloth should be thoroughly soaked in it and then wrung out. As for poultices, first rub a little oil on the area to prevent sticking, and then apply the cloth to the skin. To retain the moisture, cover the compress with plastic wrap or a plastic bag, and secure it with a bandage. Replace the compress as needed.

### COOLING COMPRESS
*200 ml (8 fl oz) lavender infusion*
*A lavender compress can be placed on the forehead or the back of the neck to relieve tension and headaches.*

*Use a cool poultice or compress for hot, inflamed conditions and a warm application to relieve strain and aching in cold, painful areas.*

## POULTICES

A poultice is a means of applying a herb to a particular area of the body. You can use the herbs in fresh, dried or powdered form.

### FRESH HERB POULTICE

First, apply a little sunflower or vegetable oil to the skin to prevent sticking. Crush the plant and place it directly on the affected area. Hold the poultice in place with a dressing or bandage.

### DRIED HERB POULTICE

Dried herbs must first be decocted by placing them in a pan with water and simmering them for approximately 5 minutes. Allow the mixture to cool. Squeeze out the liquid and keep the remaining material. Since this poultice is more difficult to apply directly, first spread the herbs evenly on the dressing.

### POWDERED HERB POULTICE

First mix the powders with a cold liquid, either water or a tincture. Stir until a fine paste is created, then spread on the dressing as described above.

# PESSARIES AND SUPPOSITORIES

❧

*Pessaries and suppositories can help relieve localized conditions,*

*such as vaginal candida, thrush and haemorrhoids. They can also*

*be used to give a herbal remedy that will be broken down by digestion*

*before it reaches the target area.*

### Method 1
*9 g (½ oz) beeswax*
*40 g (1½ oz) grated cocoa butter*
*100 ml (4 fl oz) oil*
*7 drops essential oil*

Prepare a pessary mould (available from specialist suppliers) by brushing it thinly with soft soap to prevent sticking. (If the mould is placed in the freezer beforehand, the mixture will set more quickly.) Using a double boiler, melt the beesewax in the oil, then add the cocoa butter and stir until dissolved. Remove from the heat, add the essential oil, and pour into the mould. Place in the freezer for 5 to 10 minutes, complete the setting process by putting the mould in the refrigerator. When set, cut it into pellets 2.5 cm (1 in) long .

### Method 2
*10 parts gelatin*
*15 parts glycerine*
*40 parts water-base*

The ratio of this formula is always the same, that is, 10 teaspoons, 15 teaspoons and 40 teaspoons, and so on. Soak the gelatin in the water, then dissolve over a very low heat. Add the glycerine and place in a double boiler. Allow the water to evaporate slowly until the required consistency is reached. Pour into a mould and follow the instructions given above.

### HAEMORRHOID SUPPOSITORIES
*10 parts gelatin*
*15 parts glycerin*
*40 parts witch hazel infusion*
*The astringent qualities of witch hazel will help to shrink and relieve painful haemorrhoids.*

*Pessaries and suppositories allow herbs to be absorbed into the blood directly and so to be utilized by the body. Keep them refrigerated, since they will melt at body temperature.*

# CHINESE HERBAL DECOCTIONS

*Tang means literally 'soup'; it translates as decoction, and this is one of the most common ways of taking traditional Chinese herbal medicine. With a decoction, it is possible to create a prescription made from eight to ten herbs which is carefully balanced in its properties and is directed to a specific area of the body.*

Chinese herbal decoctions generally use a greater number of herbs than Western herbal decoctions. Because the preparation of a decoction takes some time, and the cooking smell fills the house, many people prefer to use herbal tablets. However, if you wish to make your own decoctions, the guidelines below will help.

### QUANTITIES

Use approximately 750 ml (1½ pints) water with 40 g (1½ oz) of Chinese herbs. This will allow several herbs to be used in one decoction. The common dosage is 3–9 g (⅛–½ oz) per herb daily, but take note of the dosages recommended for individual herbs in the Herbal Directory. Children, the elderly, pregnant women, and those with weak digestive systems must take the smaller dosage. If a Chinese herbalist includes many herbs in a prescription, a daily dosage of 80–120 g (3–4½ oz) may be given.

### PREPARATION

There is a variety of ways of preparing a decoction, depending on the herbs used and the practitioner prescribing them. Always use a non-aluminum pot. Soak the herbs for two hours in enough water to cover them completely. Tonic herbs, such as astragalus (*huang qi*), Chinese angelica (*dang gui*), and liquorice (*gan cao*), which are used to strengthen the system, should be simmered gently in a covered pot for one hour. Herbs for more acute conditions, such as chrysanthemum (*ju hua*), burdock (*nui bang zi*), dandelion (*pu gong ying*) and honeysuckle (*jin yin hua*), should be simmered for 20–30 minutes. Strain the liquid from the herbs and drink it warm in equal doses, morning and evening.

Several Chinese herbs mentioned in this book need to be prepared differently. The volatile oils, which give these herbs their fragrance, are part of their healing qualities. Because they are easily destroyed by over-cooking, peppermint (*bo he*) and perilla leaf (*zi su ye*) should be added only in the last 5 minutes of preparation.

### GINSENG

Ginseng is another Chinese herb that is often prepared separately because of its expense. A piece of good ginseng root is worth a great deal of money and is highly valued in China for its life-enhancing properties. Put 1–9 g (1⁄16–½ oz) ginseng in a small amount of water placed over a double boiler. Simmer for an hour, then strain off the liquid. Add this to the liquid from other herbal decoctions, or drink it on its own. The ginseng root can be cooked in this way several times to extract all the benefit and to use it economically.

# CHINESE PATENT FORMULAS

*Chinese patent formulas are classical herbal prescriptions that can be taken in pill or tincture form. For this reason, they are easier to take than decoctions and consequently have increased in popularity. These traditional formulas can be an effective treatment for a wide range of ailments.*

Traditional Chinese patent formulas are still imported from China by most suppliers of Chinese herbs. Many Western manufacturers have adapted the traditional formulas to treat modern Western conditions. The Western adaptations often list the traditional formula on which the prescription is based, which is a handy reference to some of the more commonly available prescriptions.

## THE CHINESE COURT

The classical Chinese herbal formulas, which have been used for many centuries, were often known by the titles of members of the Chinese court. These formulas consist of many herbs which work in balance and harmony. The Four Gentlemen Decoction (*Si Jun Zi Tang*), was derived from the Confucian term meaning an exemplary person, and the number four, whose nature is harmonious. The chief herb, also known as the emperor, or *jun* herb, is ginseng, which strengthens the *qi*, or energy, of the body. The minister, or *chen* herb, white atractylodis rhizome (*bai zhu*), acts as the advisor, and works synergistically. The assistant, or *zuo* herb, is poria (*fu ling*), which works to balance the cloying nature of the tonic herbs to make them more digestible. The envoy, or *shi* herb, honey-fried liquorice (*zhi gan cao*), delivers the whole prescription to the digestive system and the twelve main channels of the body.

## WOMEN'S PRECIOUS PILLS (BA ZHEN WAN)

This is an excellent women's tonic which combines two classical formulas: the Four Gentlemen, which strengthens the *qi*, or energy, and the Four Substances, which nourishes the blood. It is useful in conditions of tiredness, dizziness, scanty periods, irregular menstruation, poor circulation and in the recovery from childbirth or long-term illness. It contains the herbs listed in the Four Gentlemen Decoction and Chinese angelica (*dang gui*), one of the herbs in the Four Substances, which strengthens the blood and improves circulation. Take five pills, two or three times a day.

## NOSE INFLAMMATION PILLS (BI YAN PIAN)

A useful formula for symptoms related to allergies such as sneezing, itching eyes and congested sinuses; it is also an excellent remedy for the relief of hayfever. It contains chrysanthemum flower (*ju hua*) and forsythia (*lian qiao*), which help to clear the first signs of a cold. Take four tablets, three times a day, half an hour after a meal.

### CENTRAL QI PILLS (BU ZHONG YI QI WAN)

A useful formula which helps to strengthen and invigorate the digestion. It relieves symptoms of bloating, pain, wind and alternating constipation and diarrhoea. It also helps to raise the *yang*, or lift prolapses of the uterus and rectum, and to treat haemorrhoids and varicose veins. It contains the Chinese herbs codonopsis root (*dang shen*) – which is a less-expensive substitute for ginseng – astragalus (*huang qi*), angelica (*dang gui*), and liquorice (*gan cao*), all of which help to support the immune system and strengthen the digestion. This is aided by citrus peel (*chen pi*) and ginger (*sheng jiang*) which facilitate the movement of food through the system. Take five pills, two or three times a day.

*Chinese herbal patent remedies, based on traditional Chinese formulas, are a simple way of taking herbal treatments.*

### DECOCTION FOR FRIGID EXTREMITIES (DANG GUI SI NI TANG)

Used to warm the extremities and nourish the blood, this formula is often taken in tincture form because alcohol is warming and easily absorbed into the bloodstream. It is useful in conditions of poor circulation, rheumatoid arthritis with cold symptoms, Raynaud's disease and frostbite. It contains Chinese angelica (*dang gui*), which strengthens the blood and improves the circulation, and cinnamon (*gui zhi*), which is warming. It should be used with caution, in spring and summer in warm climates, or with symptoms of heat, such as fever and sweating. Take one teaspoonful in warm water, three times a day.

### ANGELICA AND LORANTHUS PILL (DU HUO JI SHENG WAN)

A formula used to strengthen the back and lower extremities and to ease stiffness. It is helpful with low-back pain, sciatica and arthritis, especially when the condition is helped by heat and warmth, or is due to deficiency. It contains Chinese angelica (*dang gui*), which encourages circulation, and the warming herbs ginger (*sheng jiang*) and the inner bark of the cinnamon tree (*rou gui*). Take five pills, two or three times a day.

### EAR-RINGING LEFT LOVING PILLS (ER LONG ZUO CI WAN)

A variation of *Liu Wei Di Huang Wan* (*see* below), these pills help to ease symptoms of tinnitus, headache, high blood pressure, insomnia, thirst and eye pressure and irritation. Take five pills, three times a day; they can be taken as a long-term treatment.

## SIX-FLAVOUR REHMANNIA PILL (LIU WEI DI HUANG WAN)

This is a classic Chinese herbal prescription, which forms the basis for other prescriptions. It is nourishing for the *yin* aspect, strengthening the liver, kidneys and spleen. It helps to ease symptoms of weakness or pain in the lower back, burning in the palms or soles of the feet, mild night sweats, dizziness, tinnitus and a mild, constant sore throat. It can help high blood pressure and diabetes, but professional advice should first be sought. Take five pills, three times a day. These may be taken over a period of time, but may aggravate catarrhal conditions.

## BRIGHT EYES REHMANNIA PILLS (MING MU DI HUANG WAN)

A variation of *Liu Wei Di Huang Wan* which helps to benefit many eye complaints, especially in the elderly. This formula contains Chinese angelica (*dang gui*), which helps to nourish the blood and improve circulation. The herbs chrysanthemum flower (*ju hua*) and lycium fruit (*gou qi zi*) are particularly beneficial for the eyes. Take five pills, three times a day.

## LYCIUM, CHRYSANTHEMUM, REHMANNIA PILLS (QI JU DI HUANG WAN)

Another variation of *Liu Wei Di Huang Wan*, which helps to treat blurred vision, poor night vision, dry and painful eyes and pressure behind the eyes. It differs from *Ming Mu Di Huang Wan* (see above) in that it also treats headache, dizziness, irritability, restlessness and insomnia. It can be helpful with menopausal symptoms. As stated in its English name,

this formula contains lycium fruit (*gou qi zi*) and chrysanthemum flower (*ju hua*), which help to nourish the eyes. Take five pills, three times a day.

## CLEAN AIR TEA (QING QI HUA TAN WAN)

A useful prescription for the treatment of asthma, chronic bronchitis or sinus infection, when there is a thick, sticky phlegm that is difficult to clear. Take five pills, three times a day.

## MORUS, CHRYSANTHEMUM MEDICINE PILL (SANG JU YIN PIAN)

A useful pill to clear the first signs of a cough, especially a dry one, accompanied by a dry, sore throat, sneezing, runny nose and watering eyes. It contains forsythia fruit (*lian qiao*), chrysanthemum flower (*ju hua*) and peppermint (*bo he*), all of which help to eliminate symptoms of colds and flu. Take three tablets, two or three times a day.

## CODONOPSIS, PORIA, ATRACTYLODES FORMULA (SHEN LING BAI ZHU PIAN)

A useful formula for strengthening weak digestion. It helps to clear symptoms of bloating, indigestion and loose stools. It is a good tonic for children with poor appetite and slow growth. Take five pills, three times a day. Children can take three pills, two or three times a day.

## ZIZYPHUS SEED SOUP TABLET (SUAN ZAO REN TANG PIAN)

A prescription to calm the *shen* or 'spirit of the heart', helping with problems of insomnia, restlessness, heart palpitations and mental agitation. Take two tablets, three times a day.

## HEAVENLY KING BENEFIT HEART PILL (TIAN WANG BU XIN WAN)

Useful to calm the *shen* in cases where there is a deficiency or chronic tiredness. It is helpful with insomnia, anxiety, palpitations and vivid dreaming. It is also used in treating a hyperactive thyroid. Take five pills, three times a day.

## FREE AND EASY WANDERER (XIAO YAO WAN)

A basic formula used to nourish the blood, move the *qi*, or energy, and strengthen the digestion. It is helpful with a range of symptoms, such as bloating and fullness in the abdomen, menstrual disorders and tension headaches. This contains Chinese angelica (*dang gui*), which is useful for many menstrual problems. Take five pills, three times a day.

## LONICERA, FORSYTHIA DISPEL HEAT TABLETS (YIN QIAO JIE DU PIAN)

An excellent remedy to clear colds when taken at the appearance of the first symptoms, such as a sore throat, fever with chills, stiff muscles and sneezing. This formula contains the following herbs used to dispel early symptoms of colds: peppermint (*bo he*), forsythia fruit (*lian qiao*), honeysuckle (*jin yin hua*) and burdock seed (*nui bang zi*). Take five pills, every three hours for the first nine hours, then every five hours as needed. Discontinue after three days.

# THE BODY & HOW TO TREAT IT

*This section describes the different systems of the body and their related ailments. Herbal treatments and methods of application are suggested so that common complaints can be treated gently but effectively.*

# HEALING HERBS

*The ability to heal ourselves, to restore and revitalize our life force, or qi, lies within us. Plants offer simple remedies to help enhance our own healing process. Understanding how our body works helps us to appreciate its efficiency and ability to repair itself. We need to work with our body, not against it. Herbal medicine will help to support us so that we can bring about a deeper, permanent change within ourselves.*

## HOW TO USE THIS SECTION

This section covers the different systems in the body and their related ailments. Within each system there will be a brief description of how it works, its interaction with the rest of the body, and how it is viewed in terms of Chinese medicine. Suggestions for preventing illnesses and complaints will also be given, including changes in diet, lifestyle and outlook on life. Understanding the whole picture of your particular ailment will help the herbal healing process.

### CHOOSING THE RIGHT HERBS FOR THE RIGHT TREATMENT

With most ailments, several suggestions for herbal treatment will be given. These will include combinations of herbs, Chinese remedies, and external herbal treatments. Before using any herbs, please check the Herbal Directory to find out more about the herb, and take care to note any cautions, contraindications and dosages. Then read the Herbal Methods section to find out the most beneficial way of preparing the herb. If the specific dosages have not been given in the Herbal Directory, use the recommended dosages listed here. Be sure to take into account any changes in dosage for both the elderly and children.

### CAUTIONS AND CONTRAINDICATIONS

Herbs are safe to use if taken in the right amount, with cautions and contraindications observed. There is much debate about herbal safety, and we have listed precautions we have found while researching this book. Pregnancy is one condition where care needs to be taken when using herbs. Digestive problems, skin complaints and blood pressure may be aggravated by the use of certain herbs, so please check the Herbal Directory beforehand. Care must also be taken with essential oils; they should not be taken internally or used for babies. Please read the Herbal Directory carefully and seek advice from a professional herbalist if you have any doubts about the use of an herb.

## COMBINING HERBS AND DRUGS

If you are taking medication for a serious medical problem, it is best to seek advice from a professional medical herbalist and your doctor. Herbs can be used with most medications, but it is important to select the most appropriate ones. **DO NOT STOP TAKING ANY MEDICATION** without the advice of your doctor and herbalist. Be aware that taking herbs may change your need for medication, and this must be monitored regularly. For example, hawthorn berries must not be taken with certain cardiovascular medication since they will alter this, which can affect the heart.

## WHEN HERBS ARE INEFFECTIVE

Herbal treatment will vary with different types of conditions. Acute infections, such as colds and flu, will need a treatment that has an immediate effect, while chronic conditions such as arthritis will need long-term treatment. Generally, you will know in a matter of days whether an acute infection is clearing, since the symptoms will become better quickly. If one herb does not work, try some of the other herbs mentioned. If no herbal treatments seem to be effective, it is probably time to call a doctor, since symptoms of acute infections

*A balanced diet, regular physical exercise, and a positive attitude help to keep us healthy. Herbal medicine supports our natural flow of energy helping to gently heal us.*

such as fever, vomiting or diarrhoea can be debilitating and dangerous if left for more than a few days. With chronic conditions it is sometimes hard to know if the herbs are helping, since the symptoms may vary from day to day. Herbal treatment may be needed over a period of several weeks, and diet and lifestyle may also require changes. If the condition generally has not improved after several weeks, you may need to go to a professional herbalist to find the right herbs.

## HOME CARE AND PROFESSIONAL HERBALISM

Most of the herbal suggestions in this book are safe to use as a way of

looking after ourselves, our families, and friends. Herbal baths, vapourizers and simple herbal teas can be taken as part of a daily routine that helps maintain good health and feelings of well-being. There may be times when you need professional advice from a herbalist because the condition is too serious for treatment to be undertaken without experience and training. Make sure that you go to a herbalist who is registered with a recognized professional body or institute. The herbalist will take a case history and prescribe appropriate herbs; he or she will also be supportive in helping you make any other changes that are necessary.

# RESPIRATION

*We can survive only a few minutes without breathing. The air we breathe*

*brings us the essential element that is vital for life: oxygen. Our*

*respiratory system needs to be in good working order to take in revitalizing*

*oxygen and filter out the toxins that are now so much part of our environment.*

Our first contact with air is through the nose and mouth. Our nose alerts us to the smell of the air – is it fresh and fragrant, or full of toxic fumes? Sometimes we can even taste the poisonous gases in the air, and our reaction may be to hold our breath for several seconds. Infectious bacteria from someone who is ill also pass through the air. The nose, mouth and throat are our first line of defence. They contain cilia, or tiny hairs, that cleanse the nose and throat by drawing mucus and saliva into the stomach, where it is sterilized. Saliva and mucus protect the delicate lining of the mouth and nose by trapping invasive particles. In healthy surroundings these mechanisms work very well to keep us free from illness.

### THE BREATHING PROCESS

Air passes into the lungs through the bronchial tubes. Mucus and cilia in the bronchi and lungs help to keep the lungs clear. They do this by sweeping out any unwanted particles. Oxygen is absorbed into the bloodstream in the lungs, and is then carried by the circulatory system into every cell of the body to help release the

energy stored in the blood. The waste product of this process is carbon dioxide, which is brought back to the lungs and exhaled. We breathe in and out about ten to fifteen times a minute, without having to make a conscious effort. This is enough to blow up several thousand balloons a day.

### SMOKING AND POLLUTION

What we breathe becomes a part of us. Cigarette smoke and car fumes are irritants which affect people who suffer from respiratory conditions such as asthma and hayfever. Smoking also contributes to many chronic lung conditions, such as lung cancer and emphysema. High levels of

## How respiration works

*The respiratory system is responsible for introducing oxygen into the blood, which carries it to the tissues, and for removing carbon dioxide from the blood.*

*A steam inhalation of thyme opens nasal cavities.*

*Larynx (responsible for voice production). A sage gargle soothes sore throats.*

Trachea

Bronchi

Lungs
*Coltsfoot syrup helps to calm coughs.*

pollution in our cities and smoking in the home affect the onset of respiratory diseases in children. There has been an alarming rise in the number of asthmatic children who are dependent on daily doses of steroids in order to breathe.

### PREVENTION OF RESPIRATORY DISEASE

Our lifestyle has become more sedentary, and it is now necessary to make an effort to exercise. Children, especially, need to be able to run around in the fresh air – something that is becoming more difficult for them to do with the increase in pollution. Exercise can, however, help to strengthen our lungs. Aerobic exercise forces us to breathe more deeply and fully as the demand for oxygen is increased in the body. Yoga and meditation focus specifically on the way we breathe, helping us to be aware of the expansion and relaxation of the muscles in our chests so that our breathing is less constricted.

### THE CHINESE MEDICINE APPROACH

In Chinese medicine, good, strong, healthy lungs are linked with a strong protective *qi*, or energy. Our lungs help us to fight off viruses and infections before they take hold in the body. The Chinese philosophy is that we receive inspiration through the air we breathe. The lung is related to the metal element, the season of autumn (when a lot of people come down with colds), the colour white, and the emotion of grief. According to an old Chinese saying, catarrh is unshed tears.

### AILMENTS

Ailments affecting the respiratory system are very common. Often these complaints are treated with antibiotics. Herbal remedies can sometimes offer an effective alternative treatment, especially if they are taken at the first signs of illness. In this section, remedies for colds,

*The lungs help to filter the air we breathe, allowing fresh oxygen into the bloodstream and protecting us from pollutants. Higher incidences of asthma and other lung diseases can be related to cigarette smoking and traffic fumes.*

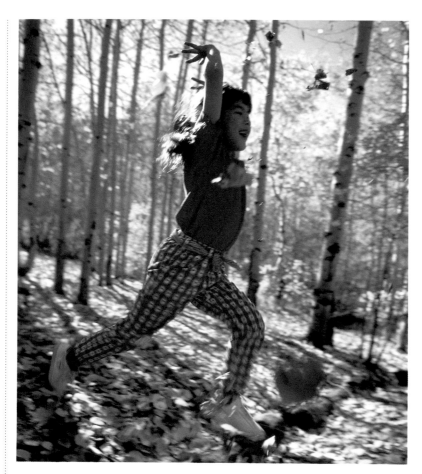

*Physical exercise helps to strengthen the body, forcing the lungs to breathe deeply and encouraging the circulation. It plays an important role in a healthy childhood.*

body. The patent remedy *Yin Qiao Jie Du Pian* is famous for getting rid of colds. The two main herbs are *jin yin hua* (honeysuckle) and *lian qiao* (forsythia). These help to clear mild chills and fever, thirst, headache and cough. It has to be taken with the first signs of a cold, within the first few days of symptoms of sneezing and sore throat, before there is a lot of catarrh. Take one teaspoon of each herb (make sure you use the Chinese herbs) and put them into a teapot with a cup of boiling water. Let it stand for 10 minutes, then drink it. Sweeten with honey if desired. Take three times a day.

influenza, sore throats, fevers, sinusitis, tonsilitis and coughs will be discussed, as well as some for asthma and hayfever.

## COLDS

Everyone has experienced the common cold. Its symptoms include sneezing, slight chills and fever, scratchy throat and a lot of catarrh. For most people a cold is merely a discomfort; however, with the elderly, babies and asthmatics we need to be careful, since a common cold could lead to a more serious chest infection. We may catch a cold when we are under stress or rundown and our resistance is low. A cold may be an indication that we need to slow down and rest. A few days off work and some herbal teas can be an ffective treatment.

### HERBAL REMEDIES

There are many herbs that are useful in relieving cold symptoms. An infusion of peppermint, elderflower and yarrow is helpful (*see* Herbal Methods section). Peppermint has a stimulating, decongestant action; elderflower is drying and anticatarrhal; and yarrow is a diaphoretic, helping to clear the virus through a light sweat.

### THE CHINESE APPROACH

In Chinese medicine, colds are said to be due to an invasion of wind, cold or heat. If our defences are low, we are more prone to give in to this invasion. If we are tired and stand in the cold wind, we will end up with a chill, sneezing and a runny nose. A fever, hot dry sore throat and catarrh may follow. When these symptoms appear, the wind and heat have invaded our

## FEVER

Fever or high body temperature is a natural response to infection. It is the body's way of clearing a virus or bacterial infection through perspiration. As viruses and bacteria are broken down by the cells of the immune system, toxins called pyrogens are released. These cause an increase in the body's metabolism and temperature. They are then sweated out through the skin. A normal body temperature is 36–37°C (96.8–98.6°F). A fever occurs when the temperature rises above 37.8°C (100°F). If the temperature rises above 38°C (103°F) and does not decrease with tepid sponging down, or if there are signs of convulsions, fits, or a stiff neck, call a doctor immediately.

### HERBAL TREATMENT

It is important to drink fluids with a fever to help the body flush out the infection. Try an infusion of camomile or limeflower, which are relaxants as well as diaphoretics. These will help ensure a good sleep, which will speed recovery. Another delicious tea can be made from one teaspoon of grated ginger and one cinnamon stick infused in one cup of boiling water, with lemon and honey to taste. This tea encourages sweating and is full of vitamin C, which helps the body to fight infections.

## INFLUENZA

If a cold and fever continue for several days and are accompanied by headache and muscular aches and pains, symptoms of flu have developed. A useful herb for these symptoms is boneset, which will quickly relieve aches and pains, as well as help the body to cope with a fever. It will also help to clear any mucous congestion in the upper respiratory tract, as well as constipation. Use an infusion of the dried or fresh herb. Drink one cup of tea as often as possible, or at least every hour. Combine boneset

*Honey is naturally healing and antiseptic. Add it to your herb tea to soothe sore throats.*

with elderflower, yarrow or ginger, depending on your symptoms. Add lemon and honey for flavour, and for vitamin C.

### INFLUENZA AND DEPRESSION

If there are signs of depression, which sometimes accompanies influenza, add skullcap to an equal measure of boneset.

## SORE THROAT

A sore throat may be the first sign of an infection. If it is accompanied by cold symptoms, use the herbs suggested for colds to help clear the sore throat. A gargle can also be made using a tea of red sage, thyme or goldenseal. All these herbs have antiseptic properties and will help fight infections. Gargle with these herbs three to six times a day. A word of warning: goldenseal is an excellent herb, but it is very bitter and should be used only in small quantities. It should also be avoided during pregnancy.

### THE PROTECTIVE ROLE OF THE TONSILS

The tonsils are part of the lymphatic system and have a protective role in defending the body against infection and pollution. They also act as a filter of poisons in the bloodstream, and of those draining from the nose and sinuses. Inflammation of the tonsils indicates an increased fight to rid the body of toxins and infections. Herbal treatment aims at supporting their work, as well as easing the pain, redness and swelling caused by tonsillitis.

### ACUTE TONSILLITIS

Acute tonsillitis flares up quickly, producing a painful and red throat.

Most commonly, it is a response to a bacterial infection. Use the herbs suggested for sore throats to ease the discomfort and to soothe the sinus membranes. A gargle of marshmallow tea will soothe a scratchy and burning throat. You should also drink a tea which helps to clear infections: use a mixture of echinacea, marigold, cleavers and camomile. The echinacea will help to boost the immune system; the marigold and cleavers support the lymphatic tissue in its cleansing work; and the camomile is calming and helps to reduce fevers.

## SINUS INFECTIONS

Sinusitis is an infection of the sinus cavities, with symptoms of headache pain and a blocked or runny nose.

### HERBAL TREATMENT

For acute sinusitis, use a combination of echinacea, to boost the immune system; goldenseal, to help clear the catarrh; and marshmallow leaves, to soothe the sinus membranes. Avoid goldenseal if you are pregnant, and try substituting one teaspoon of elderflower. If there is a fever, add yarrow to the infusion.

### STEAM INHALATION

Making a steam inhalation of aromatic herbs, such as eucalyptus and pine needles, can help to clear the sinuses. Put three teaspoons of the leaves in a basin and add 2 litres (4 pints) of boiling water. Inhale the steam through the nose for about 10 minutes (*see* Herbal Methods section). Do not go out of doors immediately after treatment, since the mucous membranes will be very sensitive.

*A steam inhalation of aromatic herbs, such as pine or eucalyptus, helps to open and clear blocked sinuses.*

### DIET AND HERBAL TREATMENT

Take a combination of cleavers and marigold as a tincture or tea for a period of several weeks to help clear the sinuses. In cases of chronic sinusitis it is necessary to look at the diet. An allergy to dairy products may cause an excessive amount of catarrh to be produced, continually inflaming the mucous membranes. Environmental factors, such as dust and pollution, should also be taken into account.

# COUGHS

Coughs are the body's attempt to remove obstruction in the throat and chest. Many herbs can be used to clear the throat and chest of irritation, phlegm, and infection, and to build up the immune system. Consult the Herbal Directory and make up a tea from a mixture of herbs to help the particular type of cough.

### DRY COUGHS

For a dry, irritating cough, take soothing, moistening herbs such as marshmallow, coltsfoot, and hyssop.

### PHLEGMY COUGHS

When the cough has loosened and is producing more phlegm, try a mixture of expectorant herbs such as hyssop, elecampane and thyme, which should also help to relax the chest and ease coughing spasms. If there is a lot of clear, runny catarrh, use ginger and cinnamon to warm it and dry it up. A tea of ginger, honey and lemon will help relieve a cough and cold with chills.

# CHEST INFECTIONS

If there are signs of a chest infection, such as fever, pain with coughing, and green phlegm, use a combination of echinacea with either elderflower, yarrow, or limeflower. If fever is persistently high or breathing is difficult, seek professional medical help.

# ASTHMA

Over the last decade there has been a dramatic rise in diagnosed cases of asthma. Many people treat their asthma successfully by using steroid inhalers. Herbal treatment can be used alongside other medication to help reduce the need for these drugs and to prevent the onset of colds and coughs, which can aggravate asthma attacks. Herbal treatment needs to take place over several months to be effective. Any reduction in medication should be done only with professional medical advice.

### THE DIET FACTOR

Asthma attacks can be triggered by allergic reactions to foods. The most common food allergens are milk produce, wheat, oranges, eggs, artificial colourings and preservatives (especially sulphur). Avoid eating one of these foods for several weeks and note if there is any difference in the number of attacks, breathlessness, or general vitality.

### ENVIRONMENTAL FACTORS

The house dustmite, which is prevalent in modern homes with central heating and carpets, is another important cause of asthma. Pets and animals can also be a trigger for wheezing and asthma attacks.

### HERBAL TREATMENT

There are a number of herbal prescriptions for asthma, and you should seek professional help from a herbalist. For mild cases, echinacea, borage and liquorice will be effective, especially if taken over several months. They all support the action of the immune system and adrenal glands, which is often low in asthmatics. Combine any one of these herbs with coltsfoot, hyssop, elecampane and thyme. These four herbs together will help to clear the phlegm and strengthen the lungs. If stress and tension are present, add either skullcap, vervain or camomile. These are relaxants, which may help the breathing to become slower and deeper.

### CHINESE HERBAL TREATMENT

Chinese herbal medicine has much to offer in the treatment of asthma. There is not sufficient space here to mention the dried herbs used, but *ma huang* is especially effective in treating attacks. This herb should be used only under the guidance of a herbalist. The patent remedy *Qing Qi Hua Tan Wan* (Clean Air Tea) is used when there is phlegm that feels as though it is stuck in the chest, causing wheeziness. It can help to move the phlegm and open the airways. The formula *Sang Ju Yin* is useful to treat the first symptoms of a cold that goes straight to the chest.

## HAYFEVER

Hayfever is an allergic reaction to various plant pollens. It is best to start treatment a few months before the hayfever season. Taking daily decoctions of echinacea or ginseng can help to build up the immune system and prevent allergic responses. Another helpful treatment is to take a dessertspoonful of honey, with the honeycomb, with each meal for a month before the season begins. Continue throughout the spring and summer.

### TREATING SYMPTOMS

Once the allergic reactions begin, a combination of elderflower, eyebright and camomile can be added to the treatment. The elderflower helps to dry the catarrh, eyebright strengthens the eyes, and camomile soothes the inflammation.

### CHINESE HERBAL TREATMENT

An excellent Chinese herbal remedy is the patent formula *Bi Yan Pian*. This formula helps to clear the nose, stop sneezing, cools and soothe the eyes, and removes heat caused by the inflammation of the mucous membranes.

*Trees, grasses and flowers can cause allergic reactions of sneezing, runny nose and red, itchy eyes. Herbal treatment for these symptoms of hayfever can be very effective.*

# THE EYES AND EARS

*Sight and hearing, along with the other senses of taste, touch, and smell,*

*help us to perceive, understand and survive in the world around us.*

## AILMENTS OF THE EYES AND EARS

Many eye and ear problems can be helped by herbal treatment, especially if diagnosed early. Herbal treatment is gentle yet effective for acute complaints such as conjunctivitis, styes, ear infections and earache. Chronic eye conditions, glue ear and tinnitus require long-term treatment, but may also respond well to herbs.

### CONJUNCTIVITIS AND BLEPHARITIS

In conjunctivitis the eye becomes irritated because of an infection, an allergy such as hayfever or pollution. Blepharitis is a more serious condition in which the eyelids become red and inflamed. Take a mixture of echinacea and eyebright as a tea, three times a day, or as pills to help boost immunity and detoxify the system. If the conjunctivitis is due to allergies, drink a tea of eyebright, camomile and yarrow three times a day. To ease inflammation, place wet camomile teabags on the closed eyes for 10 minutes at a time.

### AN HERBAL EYEWASH

Bathe the eyes regularly, using an eyewash of eyebright tea. Make sure you use a sterilized eyebath and a separate solution and towel for each eye, since these conditions are highly contagious.

### A HELPFUL CHINESE HERBAL TEA

The Chinese herb *ju hua* is also very effective in relieving symptoms of dry, red eyes with a sensitivity to light. *Ju hua* or chrysanthemum tea can be drunk regularly to help the eyes, as well as some headaches.

### STYES

Styes are caused by infection at the base of the eyelashes; they are usually an indication of being tired or rundown. They are highly contagious, so it is important to keep your towel separate from those of others. Apply warm compresses (*see* Herbal Methods section) of eyebright, burdock or marigold tea frequently during the day until the stye bursts or is reabsorbed by the body. Take echinacea, goldenseal or garlic to help clear the infection.

### CHRONIC EYE CONDITIONS

Chronic eye conditions, such as glaucoma, cataracts and macular degeneration, need long-term treatment under professional medical

### How the eyes and ears work

*Sight and hearing, along with the other senses of taste, touch and smell, help us to perceive and understand the world around us.*

*Echinacea helps to fight ear infections and relieve earache.*

*Use eyebright to strengthen the eyes.*

### GLUE EAR

Chronic ear infections can result in a condition whereby the hearing is diminished by wax and catarrh in the middle ear. Lymphatic tonics such as cleavers and marigold need to be used with herbs like elder-flower, goldenseal and hyssop, which help to clear catarrh. Treatment may be needed over several months. For children, tinctures are often easier to give. Try a diet free from dairy products for several weeks, since these often cause the body to produce more mucus.

### TINNITUS

Tinnitus creates the symptom of noises in the ear. Regular use of goldenseal or black cohosh taken over a period of time may help. The Chinese patent remedy *Lui Wei Di Huang Wan* may also be useful especially with the elderly. Or try a variation called *Er Ming Zuo Ci Wan* if the tinnitus is related to high blood pressure. Ginkgo will be effective in decreasing tinnitus for most people, but it needs to be taken for up to three months for results to be felt.

supervision. Herbal treatment, as well as advice on what vitamins and minerals to take, can help prevent and slow down deterioration. Antioxidants and bilberry will help to slow down macular degeneration and increase visual acuity.

### CHINESE REMEDIES

Two well-known Chinese patent formulas that are useful are *Qi Ju Di Huang Wan* and *Ming Mu Di Huang Wan*. They are good for chronic conditions (*see* Chinese Patent Formulas). Do not stop any medication prescribed by your doctor without his consent; the herbs are to be used only as supplements.

### EAR INFECTIONS

Infections of the ear often start in the throat and spread through the Eustachian tube. Herbal remedies that are antimicrobial and anti-catarrhal, such as goldenseal and echinacea, should be taken as a pill, tea or tincture. Garlic should be added to food or taken as garlic perles. For external use, first warm the garlic perle in your hands, then place a few drops of garlic oil from a perle in the ear, provided there is

no skin irritation in the ear canal. Use cottonwool to keep the oil in.

### EARACHE

Relieve the pain of an ear infection with a few drops of warm mullein oil or almond oil, or a few drops from a strong infusion of camomile, yarrow or hyssop tea. If there is much pain, a high fever or a thick discharge, call a doctor immediately.

*Tinnitus and chronic ear infections can result in hearing loss, interfering with the pleasure of hearing sounds around us. Herbal remedies can be helpful in the treatment of these conditions.*

# THE DIGESTIVE SYSTEM

*Our health and vitality depends on eating a well-balanced diet and the functioning of an efficient digestive system. Absorption of essential nutrients supplies the body with the necessary building blocks to keep it fit and strong.*

The digestive system begins in the mouth, where food is chewed and mixed with enzymes in the saliva to break it down. It then passes through the oesophagus to the stomach. Here, food is partly digested through the action of more enzymes and strong acid secretions that kill any harmful bacteria. In the small intestine, or duodenum, the food is mixed with enzyme-rich secretions from the pancreas and gut wall, and with bile from the liver. Essential nutrients are absorbed into the bloodstream and taken to the liver, where they are processed. In the large intestine, or colon, the fluids are absorbed into the bloodstream, leaving the residue, or faecal matter, to be expelled.

### INTERACTION WITH THE BODY

A good digestive system is a key factor in maintaining health and well-being. If the digestive system is weak or upset, we can feel tired and irritable, and be unable to concentrate and sleep. If elimination through the bowel is upset, essential food nutrients can be lost, for example, in cases of duodenal ulcers and chronic diarrhoea. Constipation can give rise to many other complaints, such as low immunity and headaches, due to toxins not being evacuated.

### THE CHINESE MEDICINE APPROACH

In Chinese medicine, digestion plays an important role in the good health of the body. The stomach and spleen are the main organs related to the digestive system, and they have the functions of breaking down the food and transporting nutrients around the body. They have a vital part in the production of *qi*, or energy. The protective *qi*, or *wei qi*, which is the basis for our immune system, is dependent on strong digestion. It is interesting that recent scientific investigations have found a strong correlation between a good immune system and a healthy digestive system.

### PREVENTION OF DIGESTIVE DISORDERS

Many disorders of the digestive system can be helped by a careful diet and good eating habits. Meals should be eaten regularly, with breakfast playing as important a part as other meals. Meal times should be relaxed. Time should be allowed to chew food properly and to allow it to be digested. The diet should include fresh fruit, vegetables and natural cereals to provide nutrients and roughage. Sugar, starches and refined flour should be kept to a minimum, and artificial additives should be avoided. Coffee, tea, alcohol and smoking should also be restricted, since they upset the digestive system.

# CONSTIPATION

*Food is broken down into a few simple forms which the body is able to utilize to provide the raw materials and energy for cellular activity*

*Food is reduced to a semi-fluid mass in the mouth.*

*Food is stored in the stomach. A gruel of slippery elm powder softens the effects of acid indigestion.*

*Food is broken down into simple compounds by the digestive juices of the gut, pancreas and liver.*

*Dandelion is an excellent liver tonic and cleanser.*

*The broken-down food is absorbed into the bloodstream in the small intestine.*

*Excess water in the residue is removed in the largel intestine. The Chinese patent remedy Shen Ling Bai Zhu Pian is very helpful for chronic diarrhoea.*

*The faeces are excreted through the anus.*

Eating too much refined food and not enough fruits, vegetables and wholegrains, which contain roughage, is a major cause of constipation. Lack of exercise, stress and food allergies can also result in constipation. In chronic constipation, the muscles of the bowel need to be stimulated to push the stools out. Long-term use of laxatives can block this natural movement (peristalsis). With ageing, the bowel can become weak and sluggish, needing more roughage and moisture to help the contents move through smoothly.

### HERBAL TREATMENT
Gentle remedies such as linseed and psyllium seeds can help to provide bulk and roughage. Soak one or two teaspoons of these seeds in 200 ml (8 fl oz) of hot water for two hours. Add lemon and honey for flavour, and drink before bedtime. If needed, another drink can be taken first thing in the morning. Linseed can also be added to a bowl of wholegrain cereal for breakfast. A decoction of more stimulating laxative herbs can be taken for up to two weeks. Use a combination of liquorice, dandelion root, yellow dock root, burdock and ginger. If

### THE EFFECT OF STRESS AND TENSION
The digestive system is richly supplied with nerves, making it prone to the effects of stress and nervous tension. The autonomic nervous system regulates the blood supply to and from the digestive system, as well as the production of the digestive juices. The digestive system is susceptible to our thoughts and emotions: as witness, we use the phrase 'gut reaction'.

### AILMENTS
In this section, ailments relating to the whole system, such as constipation, diarrhoea, nausea and vomiting, and gastric pain will be discussed. The parts of the digestive system will then be considered

separately so that ailments relating more specifically to the mouth, stomach, small intestines and large intestines can be reviewed. Herbal treatment, and some dietary advice, will be suggested for each ailment.

*A healthy diet of fresh foods, including fruits and vegetables, will provide nutrients and roughage. Good eating habits are important to help maintain a strong digestive system.*

stress and tension are involved, add camomile or crampbark. If constipation persists or is painful, seek professional medical advice.

## DIARRHOEA

Acute diarrhoea is the body's way of eliminating poisons or infections. It can occur as a result of food poisoning or stomach infections. For mild diarrhoea, drink a tea of meadowsweet to soothe and calm the gut. If it is related to an infection, drink teas of camomile, thyme, ginger or fennel, either on their own or in combination to help fight the infection and relieve ache and discomfort. Sometimes bouts of diarrhoea can be due to tension. In this case, drink teas of camomile or lemon balm combined with meadowsweet to help relax the gut. If diarrhoea persists, or if there is blood or mucus in the stools, seek professional medical advice.

*Teas and tinctures made from a combination of herbs are a gentle but effective way of easing the discomfort of digestive complaints.*

### A CHINESE REMEDY
The Chinese patent remedy *Shen Ling Bai Zhu Pian* is excellent for chronic diarrhoea due to weakness in the digestive system. It helps to tone digestion and to relieve the symptoms of belching, bloating, indigestion and abdominal fullness, as well as loose stools. It can be used with children, and is especially helpful for those who are fussy eaters, or who have allergic reactions to food. It can be used for prolonged periods.

## NAUSEA AND VOMITING

Nausea and vomiting can be symptoms of food poisoning, stomach infections, morning sickness, migraine or nervousness. To help settle the stomach, sip teas of ginger root, peppermint, or camomile. As they all have their own flavour, choose one that suits your individual taste; add honey if preferred. If there is an infection, add tinctures of echinacea or goldenseal to teas of lavender, thyme or lemon balm. If there is also stress, drink teas of camomile, lemon balm or passion flower to help you to relax. If vomiting is severe or persistent, call the doctor immediately.

### DIGESTIVE PAINS
Pain in the digestive system can be symptomatic of different problems. Any strong or persistent pains should be investigated by a doctor. Colic and griping pains are usually due to muscle spasms in the gut as it attempts to push its contents through the system. Carminative herbs, such as peppermint, ginger, fennel, lemon balm and camomile, which are specific for relieving gas and wind, can be taken as a tea or tincture in warm water after meals. Add warming spices, such as cinnamon, ginger and cardamom, to foods to ease the digestion. Massage the abdomen in a clockwise direction with a few drops of warming oil of cinnamon, ginger, cloves or peppermint diluted in a base oil.

## THE MOUTH

The digestive system begins in the mouth. Problems with the teeth and gums can make the chewing of food difficult. Treatments for toothache, gingivitis, abscesses and mouth ulcers will be suggested below, enabling the whole digestive process to become more efficient. Dental hygiene plays an important part in preventative care.

### TOOTHACHE
When problems arise, teeth must be treated by a dentist. A herbal first-aid remedy for toothache is to chew some cloves, which contain a pain-relieving oil called eugenol. Alternatively, soak a small piece of cottonwool in clove oil and place it next to the tooth. Peppermint oil can be used in the same way, but is not as effective.

### GINGIVITIS
Gingivitis is an infection of the superficial tissue of the gum. It can cause the gums to appear red and swollen and to bleed easily. Much gum disease can be reduced through good oral hygiene and by avoiding sugars and refined, processed foods. Take garlic or echinacea to help fight infections. Rinse the mouth with a teaspoon of a mixture of echinacea and myrrh tinctures in a small amount of water. This does not have a pleasant taste, but is very effective.

### ABSCESSES
A tooth abscess is a very painful condition that must be seen by the dentist. Antibiotics are the conventional form of treatment and are usually quite effective. A herbal remedy can be made from a decoction of echinacea, cleavers and poke root, which will help to

*A bright smile with healthy gums and teeth is a vital part of our expression. Good dental hygiene reduces the risk of toothache and gum infections.*

fight the infection and cleanse the lymphatic system. Garlic perles and high doses of vitamin C are also beneficial.

### MOUTH ULCERS

Mouth ulcers can indicate that the body is run down or under stress. Recovery from colds and flu, the use of antibiotics, or stress can cause an outbreak of mouth ulcers. The whole body should be treated with strengthening and calming teas of ginseng, lemon balm, vervain and liquorice. Coffee, tea and cigarette-smoking should be avoided. Treat the ulcers with a mouthwash of red sage and myrrh. In North America a commercially produced liquorice extract called 'deglycyrrhizinated licorice', or DGL, is also used in the treatment of ulcers and hyper-acidity (*see* page 122).

## THE STOMACH

The main function of the stomach is to digest food by mixing it with digestive enzymes and hydrochloric acid. Stomach acid helps to break down the food and sterilize it so that harmful bacteria are not passed on.

### INDIGESTION

Symptoms of indigestion can vary from pain and heartburn to discomfort and flatulence. They are often triggered by stress and excitement, irregular meals and over-eating. Foods that are rich, fatty or spicy should be avoided as well as coffee, tea, cigarettes and alcohol. Being allergic to certain foods will also

bring on symptoms of indigestion. The underlying cause of the indigestion needs to be treated; a change in diet and lifestyle may be what is required to bring about a long-term cure.

### HERBAL TREATMENT

With the first sign of discomfort, take slippery elm powder or tablets to soothe the inflamed stomach lining. Drink teas made from a mixture of meadowsweet, marshmallow, and liquorice, which will help to reduce stomach acid and heal inflammation. After meals, drink teas of camomile, rosemary, peppermint and fennel to help settle the stomach and aid digestion. If stress and tension are present, drink teas of camomile, lemon balm and vervain to aid relaxation.

### GASTRITIS

Gastritis is an irritation of the stomach lining, which can be caused by an infection or a reaction to food. It can start with an acute case of food poisoning or a stomach bug, and last for a while afterward. The treatment for gastritis is through diet and herbs. Drinks such as coffee, tea and alcohol, and

rich, spicy and greasy foods should be avoided. If inflammation is acute, do not eat foods high in fibre or acid, such as bran, nuts, seeds, tomatoes, vinegar and pickles. Do not smoke, since this increases the production of stomach acid.

### HERBAL TREATMENT

A decoction of the following herbs will help to soothe and heal the stomach lining. Use a mixture of one part marshmallow root and meadowsweet to half a part of goldenseal. The goldenseal has a powerful healing quality for the membranes of the stomach lining, but since it also stimulates the muscles of the uterus, it should be avoided during pregnancy. If stress and tension are aggravating the gastritis, add valerian to the decoction. Drink this tea after each meal until the condition clears.

### GASTRIC ULCER

A gastric ulcer occurs when the mucous membranes of the stomach lining break down and the digestive juices start to irritate the stomach wall. Herbal treatment is similar to that for gastritis. Take a decoction of marshmallow root, meadowsweet and goldenseal. The marshmallow root is soothing and healing to the stomach membranes. The meadowsweet helps to settle the stomach and slow the production of acid. The goldenseal is beneficial to the mucous membranes, but should be avoided in pregnancy. Take slippery elm as a powder or tablet morning and night to help protect the stomach from acid.

### FOODS TO AVOID

When a gastric ulcer forms, it is an indication that changes in the diet and lifestyle are needed if the ulcer is to be healed permanently. The diet should be low in fibre and protein while pain is acute. Eat frequent small, well-cooked meals of easily digestible foods. Avoid alcohol, tea, coffee and tobacco, as well as acidic, spicy or greasy foods. As the ulcer heals, eat a well-balanced diet, reintroducing fibre and proteins. It is best to seek professional advice for this condition.

### A CHINESE REMEDY

*Bu Zhong Yi Qi Wan* is a Chinese patent remedy that helps to strengthen the digestive system. It should not be used in acute conditions, but with more chronic complaints of abdominal bloating, pain, flatulence and erratic stools. It contains herbs that strengthen the digestion such as astragalus (*huang qi*), liquorice (*gan cao*) and ginger root (*sheng jiang*). It also contains herbs that help to move the digestive *qi*, or energy, so that feelings of fullness and abdominal bloating are eased.

## THE INTESTINES

The small intestine makes up the longest part of the digestive system – its length can be as much as 60 m (200 ft). Its main function is to absorb nutrients from the food into the bloodstream. The large intestine absorbs water and minerals. Bacteria in the gut (gut flora) help to make vitamins and to clear toxic bacteria.

### DUODENAL ULCERS

The duodenum is the first part of the small intestines. It starts below the pyloric sphincter, the valve that separates the stomach and small intestines. If it does not function properly, acid from the stomach leaks into the alkaline environment of the small intestines and can cause an ulcer.

### HERBAL TREATMENT

Make a decoction of marshmallow and liquorice root with meadowsweet and goldenseal to help heal and soothe the damaged lining. Drink this before meals. Always refer to the contraindications in the Herbal Directory before using goldenseal, liquorice, or any other herb. Slippery elm powder taken as a gruel will help to coat the gut lining and protect it from acidity and irritation. Take this first thing in the morning and last thing at night. Eat little and often, and avoid spicy, fatty or greasy foods, vinegar, coffee, tea, alcohol and tobacco. It is best to seek professional advice for treatment for this condition.

## STRESS AND TENSION

For feelings of stress and tension that often accompany ulcers, drink relaxing teas of camomile, lemon balm, vervain and skullcap, which will help to strengthen the nervous system and ease tension. Take a herbal bath with oils or strong infusions of lavender, camomile and lemon balm.

## IRRITABLE BOWEL SYNDROME (IBS)

The workings of the bowel are susceptible to our emotions. Stress and tension, along with poor eating habits and food intolerances, can aggravate any inflammation and irritation in the lining of the bowel. Symptoms of IBS include alternating diarrhoea and constipation, flatulence and

*An herbal bath with strong infusions of lavender, camomile, and lemon balm will help to relieve stress that may aggravate digestive complaints. Take a relaxing bath to soothe away cares and tensions.*

*Herbal folklore suggests a 'spring tonic' to cleanse and revitalize the body after a winter lacking in physical exercise and fresh foods. This tonic often included herbs which supported the liver.*

griping pains. This can vary from discomfort to severe pain with diarrhoea. Eliminating suspected food allergies can do a lot to relieve symptoms. Most common allergies include those to tea, coffee, milk, eggs, wheat or gluten. Any severe pain, or persistent diarrhoea or constipation, needs medical attention.

### HERBAL TREATMENT

Drink a tea made from a combination of wild yam, camomile, peppermint, marshmallow and goldenseal. The wild yam will help to relieve spasms; the camomile and peppermint will encourage good digestion; the marshmallow will soothe the inflammation; and the goldenseal helps to heal the membranes (but should only be used in small doses, and not if pregnant). Drink this three times a day over a period of time. Instead of coffee and tea, drink simple herbal teas of camomile, lemon balm and fennel to help relax and ease tensions.

### A CHINESE REMEDY

The Chinese patent formula *Xiao Yao Wan* (Free and Easy Wanderer) is helpful in cases of IBS, especially if it is worse during times of stress and accompanies PMT. It helps to relax the *qi*, or energy, and encourages digestion. It is useful to treat symptoms of abdominal bloating, fullness and poor appetite, and those symptoms that are related to food allergies.

### HAEMORRHOIDS

Haemorrhoids, or piles, is a painful condition related to the blood vessels of the rectum and anus. The most common cause is chronic constipation, and if this can be avoided the piles will be relieved. A simple infusion of the herb pilewort may tone the vessels and ease their inflammation. The astringent qualities of witch hazel, which can be made into a suppository (*see* Herbal Methods, p.31), will help to shrink the piles and relieve pain.

## THE LIVER AND GALLBLADDER

The liver is the largest organ in the body, and plays a vital role in the digestive process. It is involved in the processing of carbohydrates and is the most important organ in maintaining blood sugar levels. It helps to break down proteins and fats, and stores vitamins A, D, K and B12. The liver produces and secretes bile, which is stored in the gallbladder, and helps to break down and absorb fats, as well as activate the pancreas. The fat-soluble vitamins depend on bile for their absorption. The liver also helps to regulate hormones. It detoxifies drugs and other chemicals, helping to keep the body clear and functioning well.

### HERBAL TREATMENT FOR THE LIVER

Spring tonics, used to cleanse and support the liver after a winter of bad food, were part of folk remedy tradition. They are still relevant for the stresses of modern life: pollution, food additives, greasy fast foods, and drug and alcohol abuse all put a strain on the liver. A useful liver tonic can be made from dandelion, meadowsweet and goldenseal. The roots and leaves of dandelion make a good tonic and cleanser for the liver and the kidneys; meadowsweet will support the stomach; and goldenseal (use in small doses and avoid if pregnant) helps to tone and stimulate the digestive system. Milk thistle (or Blessed Thistle) is another excellent herb which supports and helps to cleanse the liver. Drink 2 litres (4 pints) of water a day to flush the system, and avoid eating fried, roasted or fatty foods.

# THE URINARY SYSTEM

*The urinary system has the important task of regulating the amount of water in the body and producing urine to carry away waste products. Its functioning is vital to keeping the body healthy and fit by preventing dehydration and a build-up of toxic material.*

The kidneys and bladder are the two main organs of the urinary system. The kidneys work to regulate water in the body, filter and cleanse the blood, and restore body fluids to a pure and useful state. Waste is passed out through the urine, which leaves the kidneys via the ureter to the bladder, where it is stored. It is then discharged out of the body through the urethra.

### AILMENTS

In this section herbal treatment for discomforts such as cystitis and urethritis will be discussed, as well as other related problems, such as water retention and incontinence. More serious conditions, such as prostate and kidney problems, may need advice from a professional herbalist, but some supportive herbal treatments will be suggested.

## THE KIDNEYS

Circulating blood is brought to the kidneys for filtering by the renal artery. This is a complex process, which involves the absorption of essential nutrients, cleansing of wastes and reabsorption of nutrients back into the body. The kidneys also help to maintain the acid-alkaline balance of the blood, and regulate the salt balance within the body. The adrenal glands, which produce adrenaline, are situated on top of the kidneys. They can affect the kidneys' secretion of sodium into the blood and their production of the hormone renin.

### THE CHINESE MEDICINE APPROACH

In Chinese medicine there is a strong link between the kidneys and the bladder. They are related to our energy reserves, which are frequently depleted in our society where there is a strong emphasis on achievement and hard work. The season associated with the water element, which is related to the kidneys and bladder, is winter. This is the time for resting and replenishing energy so that there will be a strong start to new growth in the spring. Weak kidney and bladder *qi*, or energy, can be related to many complaints of low-back ache and fatigue, as well as the ailments discussed here.

*Nitrogenous wastes (mainly as the simple compound urea) and acids are removed from the blood by the kidneys.*

*Blood in*

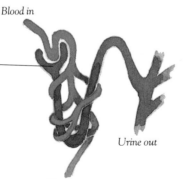

*Tubules*
*The fluid part of the blood (free of cells and protein) is filtered under pressure into long tubules in the kidney. The tubules are selectively permeable, and most of the fluid and any essential compounds are reabsorbed back into the blood. For kidney infections, drink an herbal tea of echinacea, celery seed, couchgrass and yarrow.*

*Urine out*

*Blood out*

*Urine*
*A small fraction of the fluid containing waste matter remains in the tubules and forms the urine.*

*The ureters*
*The urine passes down the ureters. Barley water helps to alkalize the urine and ease burning pains of cystitis and urethritis.*

*The bladder*
*From the ureters the urine passes into the bladder and is excreted at intervals. Drink a tea of marshmallow, couchgrass and yarrow to soothe bladder inflammation.*

## PREVENTION OF AILMENTS

Healthy functioning of any part of the body relies on the kidneys' ability to eliminate waste products and toxins. Our food and diet tend to contain many chemicals and artificial products, which puts a strain on kidney function. It is important to drink plenty of liquids to help the kidneys flush through toxins and prevent illness. Avoid drinking excessive amounts of alcohol, coffee and tea to make their job easier. To prevent strain on the bladder, try to pass water when the urge is felt rather than holding out for long periods.

# CYSTITIS AND URETHRITIS

Infection of the bladder or urethra can be a chronic or acute condition. Symptoms include a burning pain on passing urine, often accompanied by pain in the groin during or just after urination. A desire to pass water although the bladder is empty is another common symptom. Drink plenty of water to help clear the infection. Cranberry juice or extract will also help by preventing the bacteria's ability to adhere to the wall of the bladder. Take a tea of marshmallow,

couchgrass and yarrow to soothe the inflammation. If it is at an early stage, which is the best time to treat cystitis, an infusion of yarrow tea drunk three times a day may solve the problem. You can add camomile to help you relax if feelings of anxiety and tension are present. If the burning sensation is very strong, cornsilk may be added. If pain is severe, or there is a fever, seek professional medical help.

### A SOOTHING DRINK

To help alkalize the urine and ease some of the burning, drink barley water throughout the day. Use 100 g (4 oz) of washed barley with 600 ml

*Drink plenty of liquid each day to help support the kidneys' function of clearing the toxins out of the body.*

(1¼ pints) water. Simmer in a non-aluminium pot with a lid until the barley is soft. Strain and keep the liquid. Add a small amount of honey and lemon, and drink this warm.

### PREVENTION

Some women are prone to urinary-tract infection. Any disturbance within the body may start off an attack of cystitis or urethritis. Stress, overwork and antibiotics may lower resistance to infection. In this case it is important to drink at least 1 litre (2 pints) of water daily and to urinate frequently. Avoid coffee, sugar and acidic foods such as tomatoes and citrus fruits. In some individuals, caffeine will prevent the bladder from emptying completely. Deodorant douches and bathing in soapy water may cause irritation, and should be avoided.

### A CHINESE HERBAL REMEDY

There are many useful Chinese herbal remedies for cystitis and urethritis. The remedies vary, depending on whether the symptoms include blood in the urine, cloudy urine, acute pain or chronic discomfort. *Bu Zhong Yi Qi Wan* is a patent remedy useful in infections of the more chronic type. Symptoms include difficult urination, urine that comes in a weak stream, slight abdominal distension and general tiredness. This remedy is a general tonic that helps to raise the *qi*, or energy, allowing the infection to clear from the body.

## PROSTATITIS

An infection of the prostate gland is generally not as localized as cystitis and may need a more overall approach. Echinacea is a good herbal antibiotic and should be combined with couchgrass, celery seed and horsetail. As a tonic for the male hormone and gland, add saw palmetto, which helps to shrink the prostate gland. Take as a decoction or tincture three times a day (*see* Herbal Methods section). For a swollen prostate gland, take a zinc supplement or eat a handful of pumpkin seeds daily. A teaspoonful of safflower oil or cold-pressed linseed oil daily will help supply essential fatty acids. Drink a decoction of false unicorn root, dandelion, saw palmetto, couchgrass and prickly ash three times a day. Take plenty of exercise. Any swelling or discomfort of the prostate should be investigated by a doctor.

## WATER RETENTION

Water retention can be a symptom of many different problems, from circulation and kidney complaints to hormonal imbalance. It is important to find the cause of the problem, and this may involve medical tests. To treat cases of mild water retention, drink any herbal teas that have diuretic properties, the best being dandelion leaf and yarrow. (*See* Herbal Directory, page 142 for more information on the diuretic powers of dandelion.) If there is no improvement in 10 days, seek medical attention. If the water retention is part of premenstrual symptoms, add *vitex* to help balance the hormones.

## INCONTINENCE

Incontinence has both physical and psychological causes. If there is no major physical defect, herbal treatment may be helpful. It is worth a try in cases where incontinence is due to a loss of tone of the sphincter muscle, or to general muscle or nervous debility. Make a decoction of two parts of horsetail and one part of agrimony, and drink this three times a day (*see* Herbal Methods section).

## BEDWETTING

A child over the age of six who still wets the bed regularly may need medical investigation to see if there is an underlying physical problem. Bedwetting can also be due to stress, anxiety and food allergies. Avoid giving drinks before bedtime, take the child to the toilet during the night, and try to encourage dry nights with small rewards. A tea made from St John's wort, horsetail and cornsilk, sweetened with honey, will help to soothe any irritation in the bladder. Add camomile, skullcap or lemon balm if the child is stressed or worried.

### A CHINESE HERB
The Chinese herbal repertory consists mainly of plants; however, it also uses some animal parts, and even stones and minerals. For example, the Chinese herb chicken livers (*ji nei jin*) is a useful remedy for bedwetting in children. It is very effective and easy to give. The chicken livers come as a powder, which can be mixed into juice or water. Use 2 g (1 tsp) powder daily for several weeks. The remedy is also effective with incontinence in adults, and helps to dissolve urinary stones – but professional advice is needed for both of these problems.

## KIDNEY STONES

The formation of stones, or mineral deposits, in the kidney responds well to herbal treatment. A low-acid diet is recommended to help stop the stones forming; this means totally avoiding foods high in oxalic acid, such as rhubarb and spinach. Drink up to 3 litres (6 pints) of water a day, preferably one with a low mineral content, to help flush out the system. Take a combination of herbs as tea or tinctures to help dissolve and wash out the stones or gravel. A mixture of couchgrass, dandelion leaves, cleavers, marshmallow and stone root will help this condition. Extra vitamin B6 and magnesium will prevent new stones forming.

## KIDNEY INFECTIONS

Kidney infections are a serious and painful condition that need professional medical advice. The herbal treatment suggested here can be used to support medical treatment. Drink plenty of liquids, avoiding coffee, tea and alcohol. Instead, take camomile and lime-blossom tea to help relax and ease pain; drink 600 ml (1¼ pints) of the tea a day. Take a mixture of echinacea, celery seed, couchgrass and yarrow to help fight the infection.

*A large part of our body is water. Drinking 1 litre (2 pints) of water daily will help to maintain a well-functioning urinary system.*

# THE REPRODUCTIVE SYSTEM

*The reproductive system is one of nature's most miraculous 'inventions',*

*yet it can also cause anguish, pain and discomfort if there are problems.*

*The female reproductive system is mainly discussed here, along with some*

*suggestions for herbs to help male impotence and low sperm count.*

The primary female reproductive organs are the ovaries, which secrete the hormones progesterone and oestrogen and produce the ova, or eggs. Hormones secreted by the pituitary gland interact with those released by the ovaries to create the menstrual cycle. Ovulation occurs about 14 days into the menstrual cycle. If fertilization takes place, pregnancy begins. If the egg is not fertilized, it is shed with the lining of the uterus at the end of the 28-day cycle.

### CHANGES IN THE MENSTRUAL CYCLE

From the onset of the menses through to menopause, the menstrual cycle varies with each woman. Hormonal changes due to pregnancy and birth, ageing, and life events all affect the menstrual cycle. For some women this is not a problem, yet others may need some support for the discomforts brought on by these hormonal changes. Herbal treatment has been used by women for many centuries to help the body to cope with such changes.

### NATIVE AMERICAN TRADITIONS

In Native American tradition, there is a strong relationship with the earth as the mother who looks after us, providing food and a home. Traditionally, herbs were seen as part of the earth's gifts. Herb gathering was always done with prayers of thanks, and some of the plant was left to regrow. We should

Once a month, one ovum is produced. After its release from the ovary it is actively guided by movements of the fimbriae into the uterine tube.

The ovaries are the primary sex organs in the female. They secrete the hormones progesterone and oestrogen and produce the female sex cells, the ova.

The uterine tube lies folded on the side of the uterus. The ovum may be fertilized here by a spermatazoa.

Take a tea, tincture or tablet of Vitex agnus-castus to regulate the hormones.

A tea of nettles and lady's mantle will help stop heavy bleeding.

The uterus has a thick wall of smooth muscle and a vascular lining, the endometrium, which undergoes cyclical changes each month to prepare it for the acceptance of a fertilized ovum.

Vagina

Uterine tube

Bladder

Ovary

The vagina is about 3 in (8 cm) long and runs downwards and forwards to open behind the pubic bone. It sheaths the penis during sexual intercourse.

The uterine cavity enlarges enormously during pregnancy to accommodate the fetus, which grows and develops there.

The urethra is the opening of the bladder and lies in front of the vagina.

The neck of the womb, or cervix, is at the entrance to the uterine cavity. It remains tightly closed, except during childbirth, although the spermatozoa can pass through.

The clitoris is a sensitive mass of erectile tissue like a tiny copy of the male penis.

The labia are two folds of skin on the sides of these structures which hide them.

Vagina

Rectum

remember this, since some herbs are now scarce due to environmental destruction and over-picking.

## THE CHINESE APPROACH

Chinese herbal treatment for menstrual disorders focuses chiefly on the blood. Herbs are used to replenish, strengthen and move the blood, and to stop bleeding. Some prescriptions help after pregnancy, which is seen as a critical time in a woman's life. Many women have complaints in later years, which begin in the postnatal period.

## FEMALE REPRODUCTIVE SYSTEM DISORDERS

Premenstrual tension (PMT), painful periods, heavy bleeding, endometriosis, and menopausal discomforts are all related to the menstrual cycle. Herbal treatment for these will be discussed, as well as helpful herbs for conditions related to pregnancy, such as morning sickness, birth and breast feeding. Treatment for low fertility and low sex drive will also be given.

## HERBAL TREATMENT

Many of the disorders or problems related to the reproductive system are caused by hormone imbalances. Several herbs, such as ginseng, chaste berry (Vitex agnus-castus), black cohosh, and wild yam help to regulate hormone activity. These will be used along with herbs to strengthen the uterus, nourish the blood and clear infections. Wild yam contains progesterone which is useful in treating the symptoms of the menopause and postnatal depression.

# PREMENSTRUAL TENSION (PMT)

Irritability, over-sensitivity, lack of coordination, swollen and tender breasts and water retention are all symptoms of PMT. For some women they are extreme, and can start up to a week before their period is due. The symptoms are generally caused by an excess of the hormone oestrogen in relation to progesterone. PMT can also be aggravated by stress and tension in daily life. To help re-establish a hormonal balance, take 1–2 ml (20–40 drops) of *vitex* tincture, or a tablet, before breakfast each morning for several months. For stress and tension, drink a tea of motherwort, skullcap, passion flower, or valerian during the day to help relax.

### WATER RETENTION
Use teas or tinctures of dandelion, parsley or celery seed to clear water retention, which sometimes occurs as a premenstrual syndrome. Reduce the amount of salt eaten.

### A CHINESE REMEDY
The patent formula *Xiao Yao Wan* (Free and Easy Wanderer) is helpful in easing the symptoms of PMT. In Chinese medicine, the liver *qi*, or energy, helps to regulate the flow of the *qi* and blood in the body. PMT occurs when the *qi* gets 'stuck', causing feelings of irritability and frustration, as well as breast tenderness and bloating. This remedy helps to support the liver so the *qi* flows freely. Take it the week before your period is due.

### DIET SUPPLEMENTS
Evening primrose oil, taken daily for several months, can help to alleviate PMT. Calcium, magnesium, vitamins E and B-Complex are also helpful if taken regularly.

*A herbal tea can help alleviate the symptoms of premenstrual tension and aid relaxation.*

# PAINFUL PERIODS

Painful periods cause discomfort that can interrupt work and sleep. For intense cramping pains at the beginning of a period, take a tea or tincture made from crampbark, black cohosh, and liquorice (*see* Herbal Methods section). If there is tension, or the pain makes it difficult to sleep, add valerian and passion flower. Sometimes pain is relieved by a hot bath with relaxing oils or herbs of lavender or rosemary. If pain occurs each month, take *vitex* and/or diet supplements daily to help regulate the hormones.

### A CHINESE TEA
Chinese motherwort (*yi mu cao*) helps to encourage bloodflow and regulate menstruation. It is a bitter tea, but helpful when pain is at the onset of bleeding, and eases once the blood flows. It can be prepared on its own as an infusion or with Chinese angelica (*dang gui*) as a Chinese decoction (*see* p.32).

# HEAVY BLEEDING

Occasionally, bleeding during a period will be very heavy. Make an infusion using a mixture of lady's mantle, nettles, and raspberry leaf (*see* Herbal Methods section). The lady's mantle and nettles will help stop the bleeding, and the raspberry leaf strengthens the uterus. If the bleeding is severe or prolonged, consult a doctor for further investigations.

### MOXA (CHINESE MUGWORT)
*Moxa* (Chinese mugwort) can be bought in a *moxa* roll, which is like a cigar. This is lit and held over the abdomen to warm and relax the area, helping to relieve spasms or cramps. Chinese mugwort can be drunk as a tea to help stop prolonged menstrual bleeding when there are feelings of cold and weakness. It can also be used to stop bleeding in threatened miscarriage.

### RECOVERY FROM PERIODS
Menstruation can leave some women feeling depleted and tired, especially if the bleeding has been heavy. The Chinese patent remedy *Ba Zhen Wan* (Women's Precious Pills), can be taken to restore energy and fortify the blood. It contains the herb Chinese angelica (*dang gui*), which is a tonic for the blood.

# DELAYED OR SUPPRESSED BLEEDING

The delay or absence of periods can be caused by pregnancy, and this should always be tested for. Some women have an irregular cycle with no other problems, which may be a natural rhythm for them. Ill-health, emotional upsets and travel can also affect the menstrual cycle. If periods are irregular in adolescence, it may take time for a cycle to establish itself; try taking 1–2 ml (20–40 drops) of *vitex* each morning for a month. A tea or tincture of *vitex*, with other uterine tonics such as black cohosh and motherwort, taken three times a day, should help to re-establish the menstrual cycle in adult women.

## COMING OFF THE PILL

When the contraceptive pill is stopped, the body takes a while to re-establish its natural cycle. Take a mixture of *vitex*, black cohosh, liquorice, and motherwort in equal parts as a tea, three times a day, for the first two weeks after stopping the pill. Drink this twice a day for the third week, and once a day for the fourth week.

## ENDOMETRIOSIS

This is a painful condition in which the uterine lining 'escapes' from the uterus into other areas in the pelvis. Endometriosis fluctuates with hormonal changes, causing pain and sometimes very heavy bleeding. To help rebalance the hormones, take *vitex*. Use a combination of crampbark, lady's mantle and nettles to help ease pain and stop heavy bleeding. There are other helpful herbs, but these should only be prescribed by a medical herbalist.

### A MASSAGE OIL
Massage the abdomen with oils of lavender, rosemary or camomile to relieve cramping pain. Put finely chopped pieces of the herb in vegetable oil. Place this in the sun or a warm place for two weeks. Strain the herbs from the liquid, using a fine piece of muslin. Store the oil in a dark glass container (*see* Herbal Methods).

## PREGNANCY

Pregnancy is a special time. Herbal remedies have been used for centuries to help women through pregnancy and childbirth. Many herbs are safe to use and very effective; however, some herbs should be avoided (see below).

### HERBS TO AVOID
Some herbs have a stimulating effect on the uterus and should be avoided during pregnancy. The following common herbs should not be used: aloe vera, barberry, coltsfoot, comfrey, goldenseal, juniper, male fern, pennyroyal, poke root, rue, sage, tansy, thuja and wormwood. If you have any doubts about using a herb in pregnancy, check with a qualified herbalist.

## THREATENED MISCARRIAGE

Miscarriage is often the body's natural response to a pregnancy that is not right from the start, and no amount of herbal intervention will stop this. However, if a woman is under stress, or her diet is inadequate, herbs can help to strengthen and nourish her, which may prevent a threatened miscarriage. Make a decoction using herbs to tone the uterus and relax spasms. Use a mixture of 2 tsp

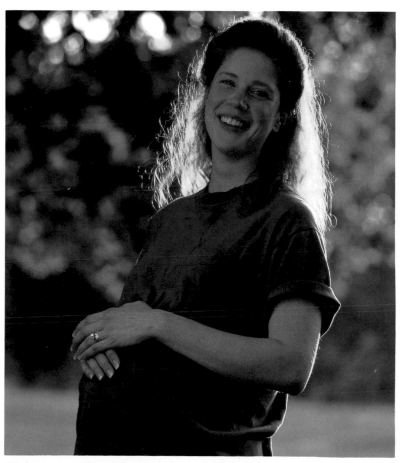

*Herbs can provide an effective and safe treatment for minor complaints of pregnancy, such as morning sickness.*

false unicorn root with 3 tsp cramp-bark in 750 ml (1½ pints) water. Simmer gently for 10 minutes and drink 200 ml (8 fl oz) three times a day. Add skullcap or valerian if there is stress.

### A CHINESE HERBAL REMEDY

Perilla leaf (*zi su ye*) is a warm and aromatic herb that can be taken for threatened miscarriage and/or morning sickness. Place 6 g (¼ oz) of the dried herb in 200 ml (8 fl oz) of water. Simmer for 15 minutes, then strain and drink twice a day. For morning sickness, add 4 g (⅛ oz) dried orange peel (*chen pi*) before cooking to help ease nausea.

## MORNING SICKNESS

Many women experience morning sickness and nausea during the first few months of pregnancy. It is frequently caused by hormonal changes and low blood sugar, so its symptoms are often strongest in the morning. Drink a sweet tea of meadowsweet, camomile, or peppermint before rising out of bed. Ginger, in the form of a biscuit, capsule or tea, may also help settle the stomach. Drink these teas throughout the day as needed. In North America, raspberry leaf tea is sometimes taken for nausea in pregnancy. However, in the Great Britain it is not used until the last three months of pregnancy (see labour, below).

*Breastfeeding ensures a baby receives the right nutrients and immunity. A tea of fennel seeds will encourage the milk flow.*

## LABOUR

During the last three months of pregnancy, drink herbal teas of raspberry leaves or squaw vine to help strengthen the uterus and prepare it for childbirth. Drink 600 ml (1¼ pints) of tea a day. While in labour, if contractions are weak and ineffective, drink a tea made from a mixture of raspberry leaves and black cohosh with a slice of ginger. If pains are very sharp and cramping, add crampbark. Massage the back and legs with dilute oils of lavender or camomile.

## RECOVERY FROM CHILDBIRTH

For many women, childbirth is not an easy process, and it may leave a woman feeling exhausted and depleted. A herbal remedy often used in China is a decoction made from Chinese angelica (*dang gui*) and astragalus (*huang qi*). The angelica revitalizes the blood and the astragalus strengthens the qi, or energy. It is especially helpful if there has been a large loss of blood or a long labour. Use 30 g (1½ oz) astragalus and 6 g (¼ oz) Chinese angelica in 800 ml (1½ pints) water. Simmer for one hour. Strain and drink warm throughout the day. Take the tea daily until strength and vitality return.

## BREASTFEEDING

Whenever possible, breast-feeding is the best way to ensure the baby receives the correct nutrients and immunity. To increase the flow of milk, drink a tea of fennel seed in combination with nettles, vervain or borage. Encourage the baby to suck as much as possible, making sure that the mother is relaxed and rested.

## PAINFUL BREASTS

If the milk flow becomes obstructed, the breasts can become enlarged and engorged. This can be very uncomfortable and may lead to mastitis, an infection of the milk glands. It is important to keep the baby feeding, although this may be uncomfortable. Apply ice-cold compresses made from poke root tea to the breasts, or use water with a few drops of lavender, fennel, or geranium oils. Place fresh cabbage leaves or rhubarb leaves in the bra between feeds. For sore, cracked nipples, use ointments of marigold (calendula) or chickweed, or rub a drop of breastmilk into the nipple after the feed.

## MASTITIS

If mastitis does set in, take a tea or tincture made from echinacea, dandelion root, yarrow and a small amount of poke root. The echinacea and dandelion root will help to clear the infection, the yarrow will relieve any fever, and the poke root will help to clear the milk ducts. Drink this three times a day, until the condition clears. Apply a warm poultice of either slippery elm and marshmallow or comfrey to the breasts (see Herbal Methods section). Bathing the breasts in hot water and applying warm compresses of distilled witch hazel will also relieve discomfort.

## MENOPAUSE

The menopause is a normal time of change and transition in a woman's life. The first signs

*During the menopause, try a herbal solution to ease the discomfort of hot flushes, depression, joint pains and insomnia. Use the herbs over a period of time to help re-establish a hormonal balance.*

may be changes in the menstrual cycle, with periods becoming irregular and hot flushes. Other discomforts may include mood swings, depression, irritability, insomnia, joint pain, low sex drive and tiredness. For many women, emotional issues such as ageing, children leaving home, and career decisions increase the pressure to re-evaluate their lives. It may be difficult to separate the changes in their lives from the changes in their bodies. A holistic approach can be supportive, emotionally and physically.

### HERBAL TREATMENT
A mixture of the following herbs will help the body to adapt to the changes in hormones, and to establish a new level of functioning. Use a combination of *vitex*, false unicorn root, St John's wort, angelica (*dang gui*) and motherwort for several months until discomfort is eased. Use 20 g (1 oz) of the mixture with 800 ml (1½ pints) water.

Prepare the angelica and false unicorn root as a decoction, simmering for 30 minutes, then add the *vitex*, St John's wort and motherwort. Drink this throughout the day (*see* Herbal Methods section).

### HOT FLUSHES
Hot flushes are a common symptom of the menopause. To relieve them, use a tea of sage and motherwort. Take vitamin E and evening primrose oil daily. Black cohosh (*see* Herbal Directory, page 114) is also useful in the treatment of symptoms of the menopause.

### TIREDNESS AND DEPRESSION
Drink a tea made from St John's wort, skullcap or vervain. Try to avoid caffeine, substituting relaxing and refreshing herbal teas, such as limeblossom, rosemary and lemon balm. Take a good multivitamin and mineral daily.

## JOINT PAINS

A Chinese herbal remedy to ease joint pains and cramping can be made from lycium fruit (*gou qi zi*) and liquorice (*gan cao*). This helps to strengthen the circulation and nourish the blood. It may also help dry skin and dryness of the eyes. Prepare as a Chinese herbal decoction using 20 g (1 oz) lycium fruit and 10 g (½ oz) of liquorice in 800 ml (1½ pints) of water. Simmer for 30 minutes. Strain and drink half of it in the morning and half in the evening.

## LOW SEX DRIVE IN WOMEN

Low sex drive can have several causes, such as general tiredness and depression, frustration in a relationship, or hormonal imbalance. It is important to understand the cause so that treatment can be effective. Herbal treatment will help with tiredness and hormonal balance, but counselling will be more effective if there is a problem in a relationship. To help balance the hormones, take 1–2 ml (20–40 drops) of *vitex* tincture each morning. Make a Chinese herbal decoction using Chinese angelica (*dang gui*) and liquorice (*gan cao*) to help overcome feelings of weakness. Drink teas of camomile, vervain and skullcap to help relax and ease tensions. Use oils of rose, neroli, geranium and jasmine in a herbal bath or a massage oil.

## IMPOTENCE

Herbal treatment to help improve men's sex drive and libido are different. A tea of damiana and saw palmetto berries will help to boost the male hormones. Add liquorice, cinnamon and ginger to warm and strengthen the body. Use oils of frankincense and cinnamon in a bath or massage. Take regular decoctions of ginseng (*see* Herbal Methods section), for up to three months, to help relieve general tiredness and revitalize sexual energy. Ginkgo will increase the blood supply to the penis. Relaxation, visualization and sometimes therapy are needed to deal with psychological impotence or anxiety about performance.

## INFERTILITY

For many couples, difficulty in conceiving can have an enormous effect on the rest of their lives. Many tests can be carried out to help find the source of the problem; medical treatment can be risky and very expensive. If there are no obvious structural problems, such as ovarian cysts or blocked fallopian tubes, it is worth trying herbal treatment because it helps to stimulate the body to heal itself. If the suggestions here do not help, try having a private consultation with a medical herbalist.

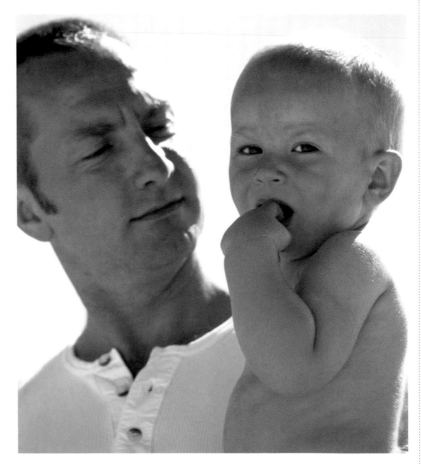

*An herbal tea of damiana and saw palmetto berries will help boost male hormones, helping with problems of impotence and a low sperm count.*

# LOW SPERM COUNT

❧

A healthy diet, free from junk food, alcohol, cigarettes and caffeine will help to increase the number of healthy sperm. Avoid tight clothing and hot baths. Take a combination of damiana, saw palmetto, celery seeds, liquorice and ginger on a regular basis as a tea or a tincture (*see* Herbal Methods section). Drink ginseng as a Chinese decoction or as a medicinal brandy, except in cases of high blood pressure (*see* below).

# DIFFICULTY IN CONCEIVING

❧

These herbs help to balance a woman's hormones and nourish the blood and uterus, so they will help to encourage conception in cases where there is no known medical cause. Over a period of several months, drink a tea of *vitex*, false unicorn root, roses, nettles, and marigold. Supplements of evening primrose oil, kelp, royal jelly and vitamin B may also help.

# GINSENG MEDICINAL BRANDY

❧

Take 100 g (4 oz) good-quality ginseng root and place it in a bottle with 1 litre (2 pints) brandy. Soak for two to three weeks. Drink 6 ml (approximately 1⅓ tsp) a day to help restore vitality and strengthen the body. Avoid using ginseng if there is high blood pressure, or during pregnancy.

## How the male reproductive system works

The primary sex organs in the male are the two testes. They lie in the scrotum outside the body cavities where they can be kept cool, as they need to be if they are to function fully.

Each testis consists of about 200 tightly coiled tubules.

The male sex cells, the spermatozoa, are produced within the tubules and emptied into the vas deferens, via the epididymis.

Vas deferens

The vas deferens carries the spermatozoa from the testis to the back of the bladder.

Bladder

Pubis

Seminal vesicles

The spermatozoa can then enter the urethra through the narrow ejaculatory ducts.

Prostate gland

The bulbo-urethral glands and the seminal vesicles add their secretions which form 90 per cent of the volume of the semen.

Drink a decoction of echinacea, couchgrass, celery seed and horsetail for an infection of the prostate gland.

The penis consists of two corpora cavernosa, which diverge to become attached to the pelvis, and a corpus spongiosum which carries the urethra. The corpus spongiosum expands to form the glans at the tip of the penis.

Rectum

Corpus spongiosum

Glans

Anus

Testis

A low sperm count will be helped with herbs such as damiana, saw palmetto and ginseng.

Scrotum

Erection of the penis is due to arterial dilatation controlled by the parasympathetic nervous system. The spongy spaces in the corpora become filled with blood at full arterial pressure.

Ejaculation expels about 3 ml of semen containing about 300 million spermatozoa into the female genital tract during sexual intercourse.

# THE ENDOCRINE SYSTEM

*The endocrine, or glandular, system controls and balances the production of hormones, which have a profound effect on the health of the body. The hypothalamus in the brain, the pituitary, thyroid and adrenal glands, the pancreas, testes and ovaries are all parts of this system.*

The processes of the endocrine system are too complex to explain in detail here. Basically, the endocrine system secretes hormones into the bloodstream, which act as chemical messengers that travel to all parts of the body. Hormone production in many cases is controlled by a negative feedback system: an over-production of one hormone will sometimes cause a decrease in another, until the balance in the body is restored. The pituitary gland plays a central role in maintaining this harmony or homeostasis.

## How the endocrine system works

*For the widespread activities of the body, such as growth, metabolism, water/salt balance and reproduction, which do not demand rapid changes, coordination throughout the body is affected by chemical messengers. These are the hormones produced by the ductless endocrine glands.*

*The thyroid gland controls the rate of metabolism. Seaweeds, such as kelp and bladderwrack, help to regulate it.*

*Borage and ginseng help support the functions of the adrenal glands.*

*Diabetes can be helped by a careful diet and the Chinese herb, lycium fruit (gou qi zi).*

### PREVENTION OF DISORDERS

A healthy endocrine system can be maintained through a good diet, a relaxed and fulfilled life, and a positive mental outlook. Many disorders are brought on through stress and tension. Because of the endocrine system's strong link with the nervous system, it may be important to take time to relax and sort out emotional difficulties. Metabolic disorders such as diabetes or over- or under-active thyroid can be inherited or occur for no known reason, but they will all be helped by a healthy, well-balanced diet.

### AILMENTS

In this section, treatments for diabetes, over-active thyroid, under-active thyroid, and the adrenal glands will be discussed. Suggestions for treatments for the ailments related to the testes and ovaries may be found in the section related to the reproductive system (*see* pp.58–65). If stress or nervous exhaustion are part of the symptom picture, consult the section on the nervous system (*see* pp.89–95).

## THE PANCREAS

The pancreas is a large gland that secretes the digestive enzymes that break down protein, fat and carbohydrates. It also produces insulin and glucagon, which regulate the amount of sugar in the blood.

### DIABETES MELLITUS

Diabetes occurs when the pancreas – or more specifically the islets of Langerhans, which are part of it – malfunctions and does not produce enough insulin. Blood sugar levels are higher than normal, and extra doses of insulin may need to be

### INTERACTION WITH THE BODY

The effects of the endocrine system can be felt in all parts of the body. It has a strong connection with the nervous system and our emotions. For example, the adrenal glands produce more adrenaline when danger threatens. This then encourages the heart to beat faster, so blood gets to the muscles to encourage their quick movements, as well as producing feelings of fear and excitement. The sexual hormones in the testes and ovaries are responsible for the reproductive process, and have a strong connection to romantic feelings. The hormones secreted by the thyroid and pancreas affect our metabolism and blood sugar levels. The functioning of these glands also alters our moods and state of mind.

### THE CHINESE APPROACH

According to Chinese medicine, the endocrine system is not related to just one other system in the body. Treatment is according to individual symptoms, as well as information obtained from the pulse and tongue. Usually, the functioning of the adrenal glands is treated specifically with herbs such as liquorice (*gan cao*) or ginseng, which support it if there are symptoms of tiredness and depletion. Various seaweeds are added to prescriptions to regulate the thyroid.

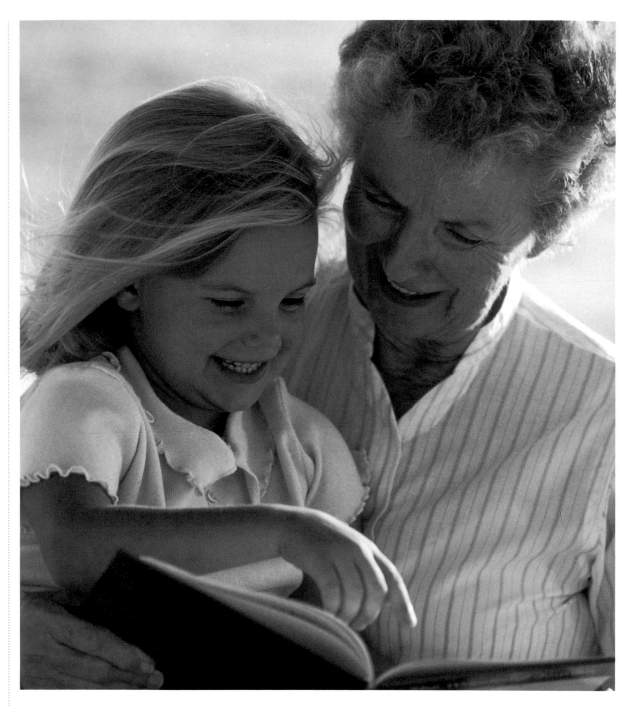

*Take time to relax and enjoy life; long-term stress and strain can undermine the balancing functions of the thyroid, pancreas and adrenal glands.*

taken, either through a syringe or tablets, depending on the severity of the diabetes. In milder cases, usually occurring in people over 50, a diet which avoids sugars and controls carbohydrate intake may be adequate to normalize the blood sugar levels. Professional advice is needed for herbal treatment. Records show that herbs and foods such as allspice, artichoke, banana, burdock, cabbage, carrot, ginseng, nettles, oats, olives, onion, papaya, peas, spinach, sunflower and turnip have properties that help to reduce the blood sugar level. The Chinese herb, lycium fruit (*gou qi zi*), can be eaten daily as a treatment.

## THE THYROID

The thyroid gland secretes hormones that help to regulate the metabolism of the body. They have an effect on the rate of digestion, appetite, weight gain or loss, and general feelings of anxiety, depression and tiredness.

### UNDER-ACTIVE THYROID

In this condition, the body's basic rate of activity is lowered, causing symptoms of weight gain, apathy and depression. Herbal treatment consists of nervine tonics and a specific herb that has an action on the thyroid, called bladderwrack, which is a type of seaweed. Combine two parts of bladderwrack with one part of damiana, nettles and oats. Drink 200 ml (8 fl oz), three times a day. Take plenty of gentle exercise, such as yoga or *t'ai chi*, to help stimulate the thyroid and keep energy moving.

### OVER-ACTIVE THYROID

This condition, in which there is an over-production of thyroid hormones, is the opposite of the one discussed above. Symptoms include over-activity, with restlessness, anxiety, tension and weight loss. Take a combination of nervine relaxants with kelp for an over-active thyroid. A helpful combination would be two parts of kelp to one part each of nettles, valerian, and yarrow.

## THE ADRENAL GLANDS

The adrenal glands are located just above the kidneys and secrete the hormone adrenaline. In stressful situations, adrenaline is released into the bloodstream to prepare the body for fight-or-flight by increasing the heart rate, raising blood pressure and stimulating breathing. Long-term stressful situations will exhaust the body and deplete the adrenal glands.

### HERBAL TREATMENT

There are several herbs that support the function of the adrenal glands. Borage and ginseng are beneficial in long-term stressful situations. Take them as teas or tinctures to help build up the adrenal glands and revitalize the body. In addition, liquorice or Chinese liquorice (*gan cao*) are used as a tonic for the adrenal glands, and are especially helpful in promoting recovery from the side-effects of steroid drugs.

*Kelp and bladderwrack are two types of seaweed that help to regulate the function of the thyroid gland. Take these in combination with other herbs.*

# THE SKIN

*The skin is the body's largest organ, completely encasing the other organs and tissues. Its many functions include protection, excretion and sensory perception. Ailments are rarely symptomatic of the skin itself; more often they are signs of complex processes involving aspects of the whole body.*

There are two layers of the skin, the epidermis and the dermis. The epidermis is the outer layer, which itself has four or five layers, with more on the soles of the feet and palms of the hands. The dermis is the innermost layer containing the blood vessels, nerves, glands and hair follicles. There are two types of glands in the skin. The sebaceous glands secrete an oil to keep the skin soft and supple. The sudoriferous, or sweat, glands pass through the dermis and open as a pore through which salts, water and acids are excreted as perspiration.

### INTERACTION WITH THE BODY

The skin is responsible for excreting about one-quarter of the body's wastes. Any problem with the skin puts a strain on the other three major organs involved in eliminating wastes, the kidneys, lungs, and bowels. Any dysfunction with these organs will also have an effect on the skin. The skin helps to regulate body temperature through perspiration, which acts as a cooling process. It protects the more vital organs from extremes in temperature, the harmful rays of the sun and invasive micro-organisms.

### THE CHINESE APPROACH

Chinese medicine sees the skin as the outer lung, which helps to explain the high correlation between asthma and eczema in many children. Chinese herbs are particularly good for treating skin conditions. Many herbs used to treat the skin are also used to help other organs to function more efficiently. Often the diagnosis is based on the appearance of the skin, as well as other, traditional, techniques. A bright red rash that bleeds easily will be due to too much heat; a weeping skin will be

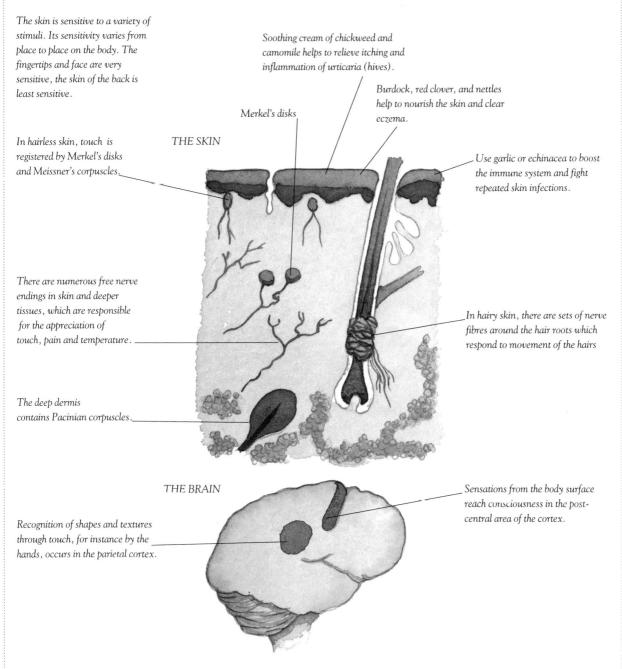

The skin is sensitive to a variety of stimuli. Its sensitivity varies from place to place on the body. The fingertips and face are very sensitive, the skin of the back is least sensitive.

Soothing cream of chickweed and camomile helps to relieve itching and inflammation of urticaria (hives).

Burdock, red clover, and nettles help to nourish the skin and clear eczema.

Merkel's disks

THE SKIN

In hairless skin, touch is registered by Merkel's disks and Meissner's corpuscles.

Use garlic or echinacea to boost the immune system and fight repeated skin infections.

There are numerous free nerve endings in skin and deeper tissues, which are responsible for the appreciation of touch, pain and temperature.

In hairy skin, there are sets of nerve fibres around the hair roots which respond to movement of the hairs

The deep dermis contains Pacinian corpuscles.

THE BRAIN

Sensations from the body surface reach consciousness in the post-central area of the cortex.

Recognition of shapes and textures through touch, for instance by the hands, occurs in the parietal cortex.

caused by excessive dampness; and dry, brittle skin will indicate a lack of moisture. The herbs employed will heal the whole body by clearing or tonifying, depending on the individual's needs. Changes in the condition of the skin as it heals will require different herbal prescriptions, so it is advisable to have an individual consultation with a Chinese herbalist.

## PREVENTION OF SKIN DISEASE

There are many different types of skin disease, which means there are many causes. It is difficult to generalize because what may be the cause for one person is not necessarily the cause for others. Some skin conditions, such as eczema and psoriasis, indicate an inherited tendency. Others, such as acne, may be

worse at certain times in a person's life. Each skin condition will need specific advice for treatment and prevention. A good diet, with plenty of fresh fruit and vegetables, drinking a lot of water, taking exercise, breathing fresh air, and a peaceful state of mind will all help the quality of the skin and the quality of life itself.

*Eating a good diet and drinking lots of water will help to keep the skin clear of blemishes.*

### AILMENTS

Skin problems vary enormously, from those that are chronic, such as eczema and psoriasis, to those that may be an instant allergic reaction, such as a rash or urticaria (hives). Bacterial, viral and fungal infections may cause acne, boils, warts, herpes and athlete's foot. These conditions are all covered here, as well as external skin problems such as bruises, burns and wounds.

## ECZEMA

Eczema is an itchy skin condition which has various forms and stages. It can appear as a red, itchy rash or weepy blisters, which then change to dry, cracked skin as they heal. Longstanding eczma can appear as dry, scaly, hard, thickened skin. If the skin is broken by scratching, it can become infected and create further inflammation. Eczema may have many causes, and it is important to find out what may help and what may aggravate it. Try to wear cotton clothing. Use a pure soap and laundry detergent for sensitive skins. Water, especially if it is very chlorinated, can dry the skin, so use oil in the bath and moisturizing creams afterwards. Avoid scratching by wearing light cotton clothing that covers itchy areas. Eczema may be aggravated by the presence of animals or by hayfever. If stress is a factor, try to deal with problems and find a more relaxing way of life.

### DIETARY FACTORS

Eczema can be triggered by food allergies, particularly dairy produce, eggs and wheat. Other foods that can cause skin reactions are citrus fruits, tomatoes, sugar, chocolate, pork, beef, peppers, and eggplant (aubergine). To find out if there is a food sensitivity, eliminate one of these foods for 10 days, then reintroduce it into the diet and observe any reaction. There may be nutritional deficiencies, and supplements of evening primrose oil, vitamins A, B, C and E, and the minerals zinc, magnesium, calcium and iron may help.

### HERBAL TREATMENTS

A hot herbal tea of echinacea and yarrow will help cleanse the blood and support the immune system. Add borage or liquorice to support the adrenal glands, especially if steroid creams have been used or are being reduced. Burdock, red clover and nettles will help to cleanse and nourish the skin. Make a decoction of several of these herbs and drink 600 ml (1¼ pints) a day. Externally, use a few drops of camomile or lemon balm oil to soothe dry skin. Aloe vera gel or comfrey ointment are also helpful. If the eczema is infected, try a bath with lavender oil, sea salt or cider vinegar. Use a compress of marigold, burdock or yellow dock on the infected area.

## PSORIASIS

&

Psoriasis is one of the most common skin conditions to affect white people, although it does occur in other races. It is distressing because of its appearance: red areas, often raised and clearly marked, produce excess epidermis, which can itch and flake off. Psoriasis often clears up with the help of sunshine and seawater. Stress, food allergies and nutritional deficiencies can aggravate it in a similar way to eczema.

### HERBAL TREATMENTS

Take herbal teas or tinctures to help relax and strengthen the nervous system. Camomile, skullcap, vervain and lemon balm are all nervine tonics and can be taken on a daily basis. Use motherwort or limeblossom if there is high blood pressure or palpitations. An infusion or decoction of burdock, nettles, cleavers and yellow dock will help to cleanse and nourish the body (*see* Herbal Methods section). If the condition has not cleared up after three months, a professional herbalist should be consulted.

## ACNE

&

Acne tends to be related to hormonal changes that occur during adolescence or at the time of the menopause. Diet can also play an important role. Try to avoid fatty foods, dairy produce, chocolate, alcohol, sweets, tea and coffee; eat plenty of fresh fruits and vegetables. Take a herbal tea made from a combination of dandelion root, burdock, cleavers and echinacea to cleanse the blood. To help regulate hormonal imbalance, women can take chaste berry (*Vitex*

*agnus-castus*) daily. Steam your face for five to ten minutes with hot infusions of lavender, camomile or thyme to cleanse the pores. Then rinse it with rosewater, honeywater, or a dilute infusion of marigold tea to tone and close the pores. Do this every day until the skin heals (this may take several months).

## URTICARIA (HIVES)

&

Urticaria is an allergic skin reaction which appears as a red rash. Sometimes the reaction can affect the mouth and lips, and in these cases a doctor should be called immediately because serious breathing difficulties could occur. It is important to identify the allergen, which is usually some food, perfume, an insect sting or even strong sunlight.

### A HERBAL BATH AND COMPRESS

To relieve itching and inflammation in acute reactions, make a strong infusion of burdock or chickweed, pour it into a hot bath and soak in it, or make a compress from a strong decoction of burdock root and yellow dock.

### A SOOTHING CREAM

Use a combination of chickweed and camomile to make a cream to relieve itching and inflammation (*see* Herbal Methods section). The chickweed is cooling, and the camomile helps to calm and soothe the irritation of the skin.

*A bath of camomile, burdock or chickweed will help to relieve acute urticaria.*

## ABSCESSES AND BOILS

&

Abscesses and boils are eruptions that are infected with pus. They occur when the skin becomes infected with the *Staphylococcus pyogenes* bacteria, often because the body is under stress or weakened. To heal these skin ailments, both internal and external treatments are needed. Use herbs such as echinacea and garlic to boost the immune system. Drink a mixture of burdock, nettles and poke root to help resolve the infection. Repeated attacks of boils can indicate that the body is run down and in need of rest and relaxation. Call your doctor if the boils do not come to a head within a few days, or if there is a fever.

EXTERNAL TREATMENT

There are several different types of compresses and poultices to help bring out pus and discharge. You can apply these for an hour or so, three times a day. Make a poultice of slippery elm and marshmallow leaves, and apply it as hot as possible (*see* Herbal Methods section). Burdock, comfrey or Chinese dandelion (*pu gong ying*) can also be mashed in hot water and used in a similar manner to make a poultice to draw out the infection.

### A CABBAGE-LEAF POULTICE

Take a few of the inner leaves of a white cabbage and wash them well. Remove the large ribs. Tap the leaves with a rolling pin to soften them and place them on the infection. Hold them in place with a bandage for half an hour. Remove them and replace with new leaves.

## WARTS

✿

Warts are caused by a viral infection, and can only take root if the body is susceptible or vulnerable. Treatment needs to be internal and external. Drink teas of cleavers, poke root and prickly ash to clear the lymphatic system and strengthen the body. Externally, apply a tincture of the herb thuja (*Thuja occidentalis*) regularly, twice a day, for a month. Vitamin E oil or garlic oil can also be put on warts to help to clear them up.

## HERPES SIMPLEX OR COLD SORES

✿

This is another common viral infection that usually takes hold in the body early in life. The infection remains unnoticed until the resistance in the body is lowered. Cold sores can be triggered by various factors, such as other infections, menstruation, stress or poor diet. Treatment includes boosting the immune system by taking high doses of vitamin C (1000 mg) daily, and improving your diet and lifestyle. Make a decoction of echinacea, cleavers, oats and poke root to help clear the lymphatic system (*see* Herbal Methods section). Drink the tea twice a day for two weeks. Externally, use a lotion made from echinacea and myrrh. A commercially produced extract of *Melissa officinalis* applied topically is also helpful in the treatment of cold sores.

## ATHLETE'S FOOT

✿

This is a fungal infection which mainly affects the groin and feet. Fungal infections, however, can appear anywhere on the skin, including the scalp and under the nails. Athlete's foot can be highly contagious, and it spreads easily in warm, moist places, such as bathrooms and swimming pools. To prevent the spread of infection, everyone should use separate cloths and towels for washing and drying. Check pets for infections, since they can be a source, and treat them as needed. Drink teas made from a combination of echinacea, nettles, dandelion root, burdock and peppermint to boost immunity. Externally, apply oils of lavender, tea tree or thyme. Tea tree oil can irritate the skin, so it is best used in a carrier, or base, oil. Use tinctures of myrrh, echinacea or goldenseal on the affected area, three times a day.

## CHRONIC FUNGAL INFECTIONS

✿

Fungal infections can be stubborn and may need long-term treatment. They can appear as

*Lavender has many beneficial properties. Use lavender oil externally to fight fungal infections such as athlete's foot and as an antiseptic for skin infections.*

*It is important to clean a cut or wound to prevent infection. A teaspoon of St John's wort tincture in a small amount of water can be used as an antiseptic.*

dandruff, acne or eczema, and professional medical diagnosis may be needed. Infections can be an indication of an imbalance in the body. Eat a healthy diet, avoiding foods that contain sugar and yeast, such as breads, cakes, alcohol, and vinegar, which encourage fungal growth. Drink pao d'arco and marigold tea instead of tea and coffee to help fight fungal infections and boost immunity. Take garlic perles and a mixture of echinacea, dandelion root and burdock tinctures to cleanse the system. Use suggested oils and tinctures to help clear external infection.

## WOUNDS

There are many herbs which help with the healing of wounds, cuts and scrapes, and also reduce scarring. Probably the most important and best known is marigold or calendula (*see* p.111). It is important to make sure the wound or cut is clean before using the cream to ensure there is no infection as it heals. Use a teaspoon of St John's wort tincture, or a few drops of lavender or thyme oil, in a small amount of water as an antiseptic. Other useful herbs, which can be made into compresses, are elderflower and goldenseal.

## BRUISES

Apply a cold compress to a bruise to help reduce swelling and bruising. To make a compress,

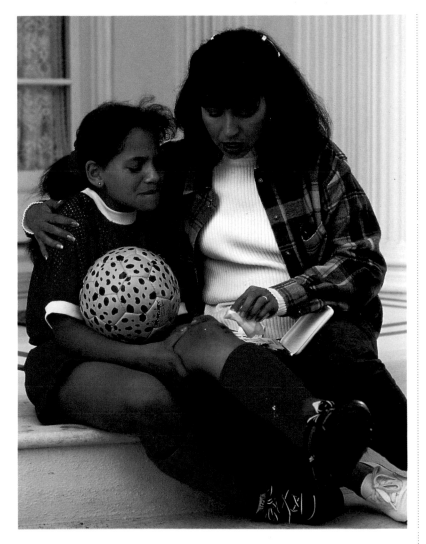

soak a clean cloth in distilled witch hazel, or in one teaspoon of arnica or marigold tincture mixed into 200 ml (8 fl oz) of water. Drink a glass of water with one drop of arnica tincture to help counter shock. Rub arnica gel, cream or ointment into the affected area until bruising is gone. Do not use arnica or comfrey on open wounds.

### ARNICA TINCTURE
Use this tincture for the treatment of bruising and sprains. Take equal amounts of fresh arnica flowers and 70 per cent alcohol, or use one part of dried flowers to 10 parts of alcohol. Mix together in a glass container and seal tightly. Shake every day for two weeks, then strain the liquid through a muslin cloth.

Leave it another two days to settle, then strain again until it is clear.

## BURNS

Immerse the burn in cold water at once to help relieve the pain. Aloe vera is very effective in the treatment of burns, since it helps to heal and cool the skin. Use it as a gel, or break open the leaf of an aloe plant and rub this on the burn. Lavender oil and calendula ointment are also effective. Use a compress soaked in distilled witch hazel, or in an infusion of comfrey, elderflower or marigold, to alleviate the pain and speed healing .

# THE CIRCULATORY SYSTEM

*This vital system transports blood to all parts of the body. The blood carries the nutrients and oxygen which feed every cell. It then carries away the waste products, which are filtered out by the lungs, kidneys and liver.*

The heart and blood vessels make up the circulatory system. The heart acts as a pump that takes in the oxygenated blood from the lungs and passes it out through the arteries into the finer network of vessels which feed the cells. The waste products are then returned through the blood in the veins back to the heart, where it is pumped to the lungs.

### INTERACTION WITH THE BODY

Disease of any part of the body will affect the circulatory system. An organ which is damaged will cause strain on the circulation. An infection or a broken bone will need extra help to remove wastes and repair the tissue. If the circulatory system is weak, it will then cause strain on other parts of the body. Poor circulation will result in cold hands and feet, chilblains, cramps and varicose veins. High and low blood pressure, arteriosclerosis and palpitations put a strain on the heart. These conditions can all be helped by herbal treatment and will be discussed in this section.

### THE CHINESE MEDICINE APPROACH

In Chinese medicine, the heart is regarded as the 'supreme controller'. The heartbeat helps to steady and reassure the other parts of the body. It holds the *shen*, or spirit of peace, which guides and directs all that we do. Ailments and remedies related to a 'disturbed *shen* of the heart' will be discussed in the section on the Nervous System. Chinese remedies for nourishing the blood will be included here. These will be helpful with anaemia and poor circulation.

## PREVENTION OF CIRCULATORY DISEASE

Prevention of circulatory disease is a far better option than undergoing treatment once problems have become established. There is a greater emphasis on educating people about the importance of diet, exercise and lifestyle. If we can take care of ourselves before an illness sets in, we will be happier and healthier. Herbal treatment can be used as part of a preventative program.

## A LOW-CHOLESTEROL DIET

Two of the most problematic foods for the circulatory system are saturated and unsaturated fat. There is strong evidence that an unhealthy, fatty diet can increase the amount of cholesterol in the blood, which may lead to arterial damage. Avoiding foods such as sugar, butter, cream, fatty meats, hard cheeses, fried foods and eggs can help prevent a high cholesterol level. Eating a diet of fresh fruits and vegetables, whole grains, and pulses has been shown to reduce cholesterol levels in the blood.

## SMOKING

Smoking is another important factor in circulatory problems. It has a complex effect on the heart and circulation which is not fully understood. It is believed that the nicotine and carbon monoxide make the heart beat faster, while at the same time causing a thickening of the blood and increasing the chances of its clotting. Heart attacks and poor circulation, both related to smoking, are serious problems in Western society.

# How the circulatory system works

*The cardiovascular system is the transport system of the body, carrying respiratory gases, foodstuffs, hormones and other material to and from the body tissues.*

*The blood is a complex fluid tissue containing specialized cells in a liquid plasma. Chinese angelica revitalizes and nourishes the blood.*

*The heart is a double pump containing four chambers, which pumps the blood into the blood vessels. A tea of hawthorn berries strengthens the heart.*

*The arteries carry blood from the heart to the tissues. Limeblossom tea clears cholesterol from the arteries.*

*The veins bring blood back from the tissues to the heart. Take garlic to improve circulation in cases of varicose veins.*

*Capillaries are minute blood vessels found throughout the tissues. They connect the small arteries to the small veins. Exchange of respiratory gases and nutrients with the tissues occurs across the walls of the capillaries. Use a foot bath with warming herbs or oils of ginger or mustard to aid poor circulation.*

*Physical exercise helps to keep us fit and well, especially now our lifestyle has become more sedentary. Smoking increases the chances of circulatory disease.*

### EXERCISE

Aerobic exercise, where the heart and lungs are stretched, helps to keep the circulatory system in good condition. When the heart beats faster, breathing becomes deeper and the blood is pumped into all parts of our body, enhancing its vitality and tone. Our lifestyle has become more sedentary; we walk less and drive more, and our work is less physically demanding. We need to make a conscious effort to exercise and keep fit.

### COPING WITH STRESS

Stress is another factor that can aggravate health problems related to the cardiovascular system. Symptoms include palpitations, chest pains and constriction, and cramping. While there are many theories as to whether stress is good or bad, what seems to be important is how we cope with stress. Herbal remedies will help to ease and alleviate symptoms of stress, but it is

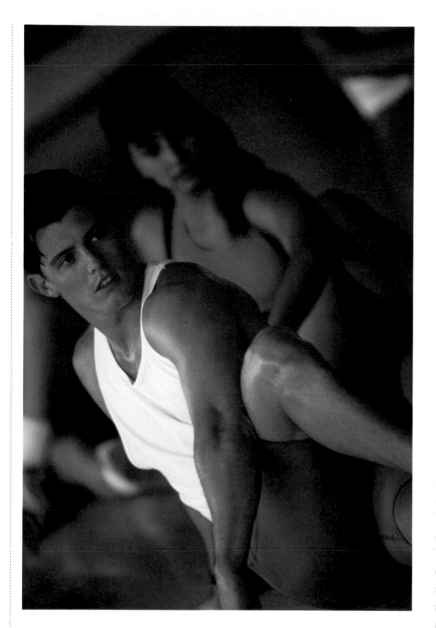

*Aerobic exercise causes the heart to beat faster and breathing to become deeper so that oxygen is circulated efficiently around the body.*

nervous tachycardia would indicate that the palpitations are due to stress and anxiety. These can be unsettling, and herbal treatment will help to relax and steady the heartbeat. Just as important, it is necessary to give up nicotine and caffeine because they stimulate and excite the heart. Do not use hawthorn if you are taking prescription heart medicines without advice from a herbal practitioner.

### HERBAL TREATMENT

An infusion using two parts of motherwort and one part of valerian makes a relaxing and soothing tea (*see* Herbal Methods section). If there are high levels of stress and anxiety, any of the relaxing herbs such as skullcap, passion flower, camomile or limeblossom may be helpful. Make an infusion using any of these herbs alone, or in combination. Drink this three times a day or as often as needed. If there is any weakness of the heart, arteriosclerosis, or heightened blood pressure, use hawthorn berries as well. They are an excellent heart tonic, and will help to normalize the heart function.

also necessary to understand the causes and deal with these.

### AILMENTS

Herbal medicine has much to offer in terms of preventing complications and easing symptoms of circulatory problems. In this section, conditions which affect the heart, such as palpitations, arteriosclerosis and high and low blood pressure, will be discussed, as well as those which affect the periphery circulation, such as varicose veins, cold hands and feet, chilblains and cramping. Suggestions of blood tonics for anaemia will also be given. More serious heart problems should always be treated under medical supervision.

## PALPITATIONS

A fast or irregular heartbeat may have many causes, and in most cases does not place any strain on the heart. Fear, excitement, stress and anxiety may all cause palpitations. If they occur frequently and regularly, it is important to see a professional medical practitioner. A diagnosis of

## ARTERIO-SCLEROSIS

Arteriosclerosis is a condition in which the artery walls thicken and harden. Initially, deposits of calcium restrict the flow of blood to the cells. Cholesterol and fatty deposits cling to the calcium, which causes a degeneration of the artery walls. They can build up in the aorta and in the arteries of the heart and brain.

### PREVENTION

Arteriosclerosis is one of the most common causes of death in the Western world. It can be aggravated by high blood pressure, a diet high in fats, lack of exercise, the excessive consumption of tea, coffee and alcohol, and also by smoking. Include foods in your diet which lower cholesterol, such as soya beans, tofu, bran and oats, lemons, garlic, leeks and onions and seeds.

### HERBAL TREATMENT

Herbal treatment includes the use of limeblossom, which with long-term use guards against the deposition of cholesterol. This can be taken as a tea, three times a day, over a period of time. Hawthorn berries will strengthen the heart muscle, while yarrow or dandelion root will act as a diuretic, helping

to circulate the blood through the kidneys to avoid water retention.

# HIGH BLOOD PRESSURE (HYPERTENSION)

Hypertension is a common condition which needs monitoring once it becomes established. It may be caused by a wide range of physical conditions, but can also have no known cause. There are several factors which can contribute to hypertension, one being a genetic predisposition. Although this cannot be altered, there are several precautions which can help to maintain healthy blood pressure.

### MONITORING BLOOD PRESSURE

Our blood pressure fluctuates during the day, depending on what we are doing. Stress and anxiety

may affect blood pressure. Often the process of taking the blood pressure itself will cause it to rise, especially if there is a stressful wait to have it done. It is important to monitor blood pressure over a period of time. Treatment in the early stages can be very helpful in preventing hypertension from becoming a permanent condition that needs daily medication.

### RELAXATION AND EXERCISE

Emotional problems and tension cause muscular constriction, which can tighten the blood vessels and influence the heartbeat. Relaxation, yoga and massage can help the body to release tension and increase circulation. Herbal baths or aromatherapy oils such as lavender, rose and lemon balm can be another way of releasing stresses and strains. Regular exercise helps the circulation and is a very good way to unwind.

*To monitor blood pressure effectively, readings should be taken over a period of time. Herbal treatment in the early stages can prevent high blood pressure from becoming a condition that needs daily medication.*

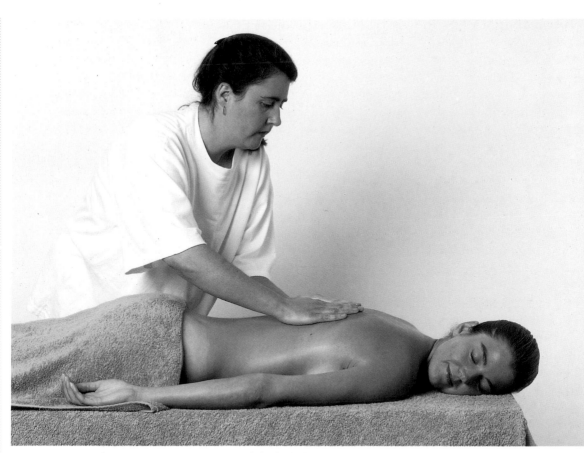

*Massage, yoga and other forms of relaxation can help the body to release tensions and increase circulation. Aromatherapy oils such as lavender, rose and lemon balm aid this process.*

### THE DIET FACTOR

A diet rich in fats and carbohydrates may be a factor in high cholesterol, which in turn may cause a build-up in the arteries. Avoid these, as well as tea, coffee, alcohol and smoking. Use olive oil, and eat plenty of fresh fruit and vegetables, nuts and seeds, and whole grains, as well as raw garlic or garlic perles. In time, garlic will help reduce blood pressure and lower cholesterol levels.

### HERBAL TREATMENT

Herbal treatment includes a mixture of hawthorn berries, limeflower, nettles and motherwort. The hawthorn berries and motherwort are tonics for the heart and help to normalize its functions. Motherwort and limeflowers are relaxants, and limeflowers are excellent for clearing any build-up

of cholesterol. Stinging nettle is strengthening and supporting to the whole body, and help to reinvigorate the blood. Make a herbal infusion and drink 600 ml (1¼ pints) a day. If you are under a great deal of stress, add either valerian, passion flower or skullcap. For water retention, use diuretic herbs such as dandelion or yarrow – add them to the mixture of dried herbs above. Fresh dandelion leaves can be eaten in salads.

### CHINESE REMEDIES

The Chinese patent remedy *Er Ming Zuo Ci Wan* can be used for treating hypertension. It will help to nourish the *Yin* energy, which often becomes deficient with age and overwork, and to clear symptoms of heat. These may include headache, insomnia, eye irritation, irritability and thirst.

## LOW BLOOD PRESSURE (HYPOTENSION)

This is a far less serious complaint than hypertension, but its symptoms of lethargy and tiredness can make life just as difficult. Take the herbs ginger, cayenne or angelica as a tea or tincture (*see* Herbal Methods section). Adding ginger and cayenne to foods can warm and stimulate the circulation. In addition, drink a tea of hawthorn berries and nettle for several weeks. This will help to regulate the blood pressure and strengthen the system. Use warming oils or herbs, such as rosemary, ginger or cinnamon in hand-and-foot baths (*see* Herbal Methods section).

# VARICOSE VEINS

Enlarged and aching of veins can be caused by too much standing or too little exercise. The condition is often inherited, and pregnancy, constipation and being overweight can aggravate it. Make sure that the feet are elevated when sitting for long periods of time to counteract the effects of gravity, and take exercise, since muscular movement helps the blood to return to the heart through the veins.

### HERBAL TREATMENT

Herbal medicine can help this condition when supported by exercise. A mixture of yarrow, St John's wort, limeflower and hawthorn berries will help to improve circulation and strengthen the veins. To ease local inflammation, use a compress soaked in witch hazel or in teas of comfrey or marigold (*see* Herbal Methods section). For severe aching, spray the area with cold water or apply crushed ice for several seconds. Massage the muscles around this area with oils of lavender, juniper or rosemary. Take garlic to improve the circulation as well as supplements of vitamins B-Complex, C, E and zinc.

# POOR CIRCULATION

This can result in cold hands and feet. Exercise and eating green, leafy vegetables can help strengthen the blood and circulation. Use warming spices such as cinnamon, ginger, cloves, chilli and cayenne in cooking. Add several slices of ginger root to your favorite tea. Make an infusion using equal parts of prickly ash bark or berries and hawthorn berries, and add a slice of ginger. Drink this three times a day, especially in cold weather. The prickly ash will help to stimulate the circulation, the hawthorn acts as a tonic for the circulation, and the ginger is warming. Garlic is also warming and helps to cleanse and strengthen the blood vessels.

### HAND-AND-FOOT BATHS

Make a hand-and-foot bath, using warming herbs or oils such as ginger, cinnamon, mustard or black pepper (*see* Herbal Methods section).

### CHILBLAINS

Chilblains are red swellings, usually on the fingers and toes, caused by exposure to the cold. Follow the advice given for poor circulation, above. It is important to protect the hands and feet by wearing warm gloves and socks. Use rubber gloves to protect the hands while washing dishes, or if immersing them in cold water. If the chilblains are itching, soothe them with marigold (calendula) ointment or oil of lavender. If the skin is not broken, put arnica ointment, neat lemon juice or cayenne ointment on the chilblains.

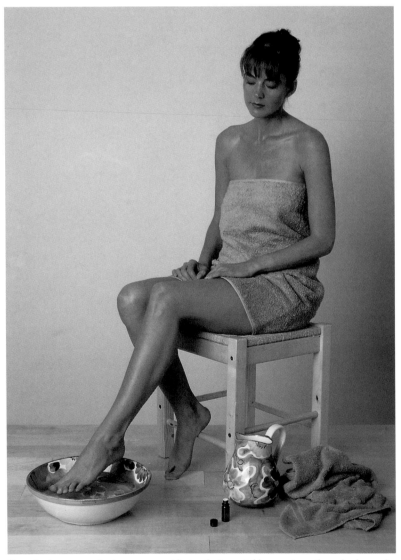

*Foot baths are a relaxing way to aid circulation. Add warming oils or herbs such as cinnamon, mustard or black pepper to treat cold feet.*

*Cold hands and feet can be helped by the Chinese remedy* Dang Gui Si Ni Tang, *which contains Chinese angelica* (dang gui) *and cinnamon.*

### CHINESE REMEDIES

There is an excellent Chinese herbal formula for warming the extremities. It is useful in chronic conditions in which the hands and feet feel very cold to the person and are cold to the touch. It can also be helpful in the treatment of Raynaud's disease, and cold rheumatic and arthritic conditions. *Dang Gui Si Ni Tang* (*Dang Gui Decoction For Frigid Extremities*) warms the channels, disperses the cold, nourishes the blood and unblocks the blood vessels. It should be used with caution during spring and summer, in warm climates, and if there are symptoms of heat, such as a red face, hot flushes or sensations of warmth.

## ANAEMIA

In anaemia there is a lack of oxygen-carrying haemoglobin in the blood. Anaemia can be caused by a loss of blood, an inherited abnormality of the red blood cells, or an inability to produce red blood cells. Symptoms include tiredness, dizziness, shortness of breath, pallor and headaches. The four main types of anaemia are iron deficiency; pernicious; megaloblastic; and sickle-cell. A simple blood test will reveal if anaemia is present. It is then important to find its cause, for which professional medical attention is needed.

### TYPES OF ANAEMIA

Anaemia caused by iron deficiency is the most common form. This can be the result of poor diet, loss of blood, illness and infection. Pernicious anaemia is due to a lack of vitamin B12. Megaloblastic anaemia occurs because of a shortage of folic acid, one of the many B vitamins. Sickle-cell anaemia is an inherited blood disorder which can affect some African and Middle Eastern people; this needs professional medical treatment.

### THE DIET FACTOR

Dietary and herbal treatments can help revitalize the blood. Eating plenty of iron-rich foods, such as dark-green, leafy vegetables, walnuts, raisins, parsley, apricots and pumpkin seeds, and drinking red wine in moderation, will help.

### HERBAL TREATMENT

Herbal teas made from chickweed, nettle, and dandelion leaves, and decoctions of burdock and yellow dock root will all replenish the blood. Drink three cups a day, using one herb or several of them in combination (*see* Herbal Methods section).

### A MEDICINAL WINE

A medicinal wine to help in the treatment of anaemia can be made with 200 g (8 oz) yellow dock, 4 g (2 tsp) of liquorice root, 4 g (2 tsp) of juniper berries, 50 g (2 oz) dried nettles, 50 g (2 oz) chopped dried apricots, and 100 g (4 oz) of sugar added to one litre (2 pints) of red wine. Allow to soak for two weeks then strain and put into a sterilized bottle. Drink one sherry glassful a day on an empty stomach. (*See also* medicinal wines in Herbal Methods section.)

# THE MUSCULOSKELETAL SYSTEM

*The bones and muscles give shape and form to the body. Their movement and strength vary with each individual and with their age, determining their physical ability throughout their lives. It is important to maintain the good health of the bones and muscles, especially as we grow older.*

The adult skeleton consists of 206 bones, which are made of living tissue that is rich in blood and nerves. Bones are living things that grow and repair themselves. The muscles account for half an adult's bodyweight; their primary function is to move the skeleton. The muscles may be attached directly to the bones, or may be connected by tendons. The muscles and tendons do not act in isolation, but as part of a muscle group controlled by the nervous system.

## INTERACTION WITH THE BODY

Muscles and bones form a framework which protects and holds in place the vital organs of the body. The bones are a reservoir of calcium, phosphorous, sodium and other elements. Red and white blood cells are produced within bone marrow. The bones, muscles and tendons maintain their strength and suppleness through exercise, and nutrients from our diet. Many of the chronic ailments affecting this system are related to these two factors.

## THE CHINESE MEDICINE APPROACH

In Chinese medicine, there are several energies that relate to the muscles and bones. The bones are connected with the kidney *qi*, or energy; the muscles to the spleen *qi*; the tendons to the liver and gall-bladder *qi*. Ailments related to muscles, bones and tendons may involve treatments for these different energies, but may also include herbs to nourish the blood and aid circulation. Such ailments are described as being 'hot' or 'cold', and cooling or warming herbs are respectively part of

*The skeleton provides a rigid framework to support the body and maintain its shape. The main function of the skeleton is to provide a system of levers, moved by skeletal muscle, allowing the body to move.*

*The skeleton surrounds and protects the soft internal organs.*

*Arthritic pain in joints can be helped by a careful diet and herbal teas of celery seed, burdock, meadowsweet, echinacea, and wild yam.*

*Du Huo Ji Sheng Wan is an excellent Chinese patent remedy to strengthen the back, especially in the elderly.*

*The individual bones are attached to one another by complex joints, which allow a variable degree of movement between the bones, and yet are strong enough to prevent the bones being pulled apart.*

*Massage the tender areas of sciatic pain with oils made from St John's wort or lavender.*

*Soak a sprained ankle in a footbath with arnica tincture to ease swelling and speed healing.*

THE SKELETON

*Skeletal muscle makes up about half the weight of the average adult. The skeletal muscles are, with a few exceptions, attached to the bone, either directly or via tendons. They move the bones at their joints when they contract. The muscles only exert their power during contraction. Several muscles are attached around a joint to permit a variety of opposing movements.*

Contract

Relax

Skeletal muscles

THE ELBOW JOINT

the treatment. For example, stiff, cold arthritic joints require the use of warming and strengthening herbs; red, swollen hot joints need herbs that clear heat and toxicity.

## PREVENTION OF DISORDERS

The health of the musculoskeletal system is affected by the way we use it. Good posture, exercise and a healthy diet all contribute to long-term good health. The Alexander Technique and yoga can help to promote healthy posture and keep the muscles and joints supple. A great deal can be done to heal structural problems with the use of osteopathy or chiropractics, especially those resulting from accidents or injuries. Emotional stress and tension can cause rigidity of the bones and muscles; these should be dealt with before they bring about a serious condition.

## AILMENTS

Rheumatism, arthritis and gout are conditions commonly found in the elderly. Herbal treatments and diet advice will be suggested for these ailments. Treatments for backache and sciatica will be given, with some herbs to be taken as teas and others to be used in a soothing herbal bath. Cramps and sprains are usually temporary conditions, and suggestions will be given to ease discomfort.

# RHEUMATISM AND ARTHRITIS

Rheumatism and arthritis both have symptoms of painful, swollen and stiff joints. Often the conditions are inherited, and symptoms occur as the result of the body's inability to cope with an

Rheumatism and arthritis may develop in later years from constant strain on one part of the body, or as a result of an accident or injury.

### A CHINESE HERBAL REMEDY

A sweet-tasting Chinese herbal remedy that is useful for easing stiffness, especially in the elderly, can be made from lycium fruit (*gou qi zi*) and Chinese liquorice (*gan cao*). Combine 20 g (1 oz) lycium fruit with 10 g (½ oz) liquorice in a pot with 800 ml (1½ pints) water. Simmer gently for 30 minutes, then strain. Drink half in the morning, and the other half in the evening. The lycium fruit will nourish the blood, while the liquorice will strengthen the *qi*, or energy.

inappropriate diet and a stressful life. Rheumatism and arthritis can be the result of an injury or accident. Constant strain from physical work may cause an arthritic condition later on, such as the arthritic shoulder of a builder who has carried bricks on his back for many years. The weather often plays a role, with the cold and damp having the worst effect.

### DIETARY ADVICE

One of the causes of rheumatism and arthritis is an accumulation of toxins and waste products in the joints, which an inappropriate diet can aggravate. Generally, foods that cause an acidic reaction in the stomach should be avoided: red meats, eggs and dairy products, vinegar, refined sugar and many spices. In addition, foods high in oxalic acid, such as rhubarb, gooseberries, and black and red currants, should not be eaten. In some instances, food allergies can result in arthritis and an elimination diet may help. This is best done with advice from a dietician. Herbal teas should be substituted for coffee, tea and alcohol. Include fresh fruit and vegetables, and drink 1½ litres (3 pints) water daily. Add a teaspoon of cider vinegar to a glass of water and drink this each morning.

### HERBAL TREATMENT

A tea made from a combination of celery seed, burdock, meadowsweet and echinacea will help to clear waste from the system. Add wild yam or devil's claw to reduce pain and swelling. If there is constipation, drink aloe vera juice, or take a decoction of yellow dock and liquorice (*see* Herbal Methods section). Take supplements of evening primrose oil or cod liver oil to keep joints supple. Rub joints with oils of lavender, rosemary, peppermint or arnica.

# GOUT

This is a specific joint problem caused by a build-up of uric acid in the body. It can be a very painful condition which often affects the feet. Herbal treatment includes a combination of anti-rheumatic herbs and diuretics to aid the process of elimination via the kidneys. Use equal amounts of burdock root, celery seed and yarrow to make a decoction. Drink it three times a day over a period of time (*see* Herbal Methods section).

### DIETARY AID

Diet is of primary importance in the treatment of gout. Avoid any foods that encourage the body's production of uric acid, such as sardines, anchovies, crab and shellfish, as well as liver, kidneys and beans. Coffee and tea, and especially alcohol, should not be drunk. Gout may be helped by taking folic acid and vitamin C supplements.

# BACKACHE

Backache can have many causes, and these should be investigated to help determine the best treatment. If backache is the result of strained muscles caused by a sudden violent movement or overuse, massage the area with oils of lavender, rosemary or St John's wort to help relieve stiffness and pain. A hot bath with a strong herbal infusion of camomile will help the muscles to relax. Use frequent hot compresses soaked in crampbark, valerian or ginger. Make a hot salt compress by heating salt in a frying pan and wrapping it in a soft cloth. The salt will hold the heat, which will help to relax muscle spasm.

### CHINESE PATENT REMEDIES

*Du Huo Ji Sheng Wan* is a patent remedy that is good for treating chronic backache, sciatica, arthritis and rheumatism affecting the lower back and limbs. It contains herbs to strengthen the body and is often used for older people. Since it contains warming herbs, it should not be used where there are hot, swollen joints, fevers, or night sweats. It is helpful for ailments that are made worse by the cold and damp.

Another Chinese herbal remedy for weakness and pain in the lower back is *Liu Wei Di Huang Wan*. It is used for conditions with symptoms of some heat, such as restlessness, insomnia, mild night sweats, dizziness, tinnitus, high blood pressure, and burning in the soles and palms. *Du Huo Ji Sheng Wan* has warming herbs in the prescription, so it is not recommended in these cases. This remedy can be used over a long period of time. (See also *moxa*, below.)

# SCIATICA

Sciatica is an inflammation of the sciatic nerve, which runs from the buttock down the back of the leg into the calf. Sciatica can cause intense pain and tenderness. It is often due to a problem in the lower back, and osteopathic or chiropractic treatment is useful. Some cases of sciatica are caused by neuralgia, or nerve pain, and treatment using nerve relaxants and tonics is helpful. Drink teas of camomile, passion flower and valerian to help soothe the inflammation and relax the muscles surrounding the nerve. Add skullcap and vervain to support the nervous system. Massage the buttock and leg with lavender and St John's wort oil to relieve the pain (*see* Herbal Methods section for a recipe for a nerve tonic oil, and *moxa*, below).

# SPRAINS

Muscles, ligaments and tendons can be pulled through accidents and injuries resulting in a sprain. Soak in a hot bath with rosemary or thyme to increase circulation to the injured area and speed healing. Arnica tincture can be used to make a hot compress or bath. Use 1 teaspoon in ½ litre (1 pint) water (*see* Herbal Methods section). Soak the sprain for 15 minutes in the solution, repeating every four hours. Arnica gel, cream, or ointment will also help but do not use if the skin is broken.

### MOXA (CHINESE MUGWORT)

*Moxa* (Chinese mugwort) can be obtained in a stick, which is called a *moxa* roll. The dried herb is compressed and rolled in paper to make an herbal 'cigar'. The lighted 'cigar' is placed near the painful area, which is warmed with it for 10 minutes, twice a day. (To extinguish the *moxa* roll, cut off the lit end and let it drop into a bowl of water.) *Moxa* can also be used to relieve back pain and sciatica. Use acupuncture with the *moxa* to speed relief.

*Lavender or St John's wort oil can help to ease back or neck pain, but professional help from a chiropractor or osteopath may be needed.*

# THE NERVOUS SYSTEM

*A holistic approach is one that recognizes the interaction of the physical*

*and psychological, with the nervous system as the link.*

*Symptoms of stress may have a physical reaction, but it is the nervous*

*system that helps us to cope with stress.*

The nervous system helps the body to communicate and control its different parts. It is made up of the brain, the nerve cells and the nerve fibres that run throughout the body. It coordinates our physical reactions, controls the involuntary muscles and organs, such as those used in breathing, and helps us interpret and react to our environment through the senses.

## THE EMOTIONAL ASPECT

In today's society there are many demands and pressures involving work and family commitments. It is the nervous system that takes the strain and helps us to cope with a way of life that is becoming ever faster and more complicated. Every aspect of our lives, from what we eat to where we live, involves greater choices and more difficult decisions than it did a generation ago. Taking care of ourselves means making a conscious effort to relax and enjoy our life. This is sometimes difficult to do in our society where neuroses can seem the only answer to its demands. Herbal treatment can help us to achieve some emotional stability in a fast-changing world.

## AFFECTING THE BODY

There are a number of physical ailments which have a strong relationship to the nervous system. These include high blood pressure, coronary disease, asthma, indigestion, ulcers, skin rashes and menstrual problems. In treating these ailments, which are discussed in other sections of the book, it may

*The nervous system consists of the brain, nerve cells, and nerve fibres. It conducts messages to and from the brain and around the body, and also helps maintain homeostasis, or balance, within the body.*

*Brain*
Drink teas of camomile, skullcup, and feverfew to relieve headaches and aid relaxation.

*Nervous system*
Rub in oils made with lavender and St John's wort to soothe inflamed nerve pain.

*Involuntary organs and muscles*

*Voluntary muscles*
Take tinctures of valerian and crampbark to relax tense muscles.

be useful to consider some of the herbs suggested here, especially if stress and anxiety are making these conditions worse.

### THE CHINESE MEDICINE APPROACH

In Chinese medicine, disorders of the nervous system are seen as the result of disturbances of *shen*, or the spirit of the heart. The heart is considered to be the 'supreme controller', and a calm, steady heartbeat tells the body that all is well. Stress and anxiety, insomnia, or hyperactivity can affect the heartbeat and disturb the heart's *shen*. According to Chinese medicine,

these types of disorder can also come from a deficiency or stagnation of *qi*, or energy. For instance, depression can be the result of tiredness, or may be caused by lethargy or inactivity. Many times it comes from an interaction between the two.

*Gardening, walking and the company of friends are all enjoyable ways to relax, exercise, breathe fresh air and, at the same time, relieve tensions.*

### RELAXATION

Relaxation and meditation are two ways of relieving stress and tension. When the body and the mind are in a state of peace, healing can take place. Even if this is for only one hour a day, it can have a profound effect on the rest of daily life. There are many ways of relaxing, including gardening, listening to music or taking a walk. What is important is to take time to forget about worries and cares.

### BODYWORK

Exercise is another important way of helping to support the nervous system. Tense muscles restrict blood flow and breathing. Whether it is a vigorous game of squash or a gentle hour of yoga, the muscles will relax and feelings of well-being will return. Massage, aromatherapy and other therapies that work on the body help to keep us supple and at ease.

### COUNSELLING

Counselling and psychotherapy can help to increase our understanding of our responses to difficult situations. Past traumas and negative patterns can hinder our ability to sort out problems in a positive way. Talking with others can bring new ideas for coping with stressful events. It is important to feel that others care and listen to us, especially in a society in which other people are becoming increasingly anonymous.

### CAFFEINE AND NICOTINE

Caffeine and nicotine are both stimulants. They cause the heart to beat faster and the adrenal glands to produce more adrenaline. The body does this naturally in a crisis so that there is sufficient energy to cope. Coffee, tea and smoking place a strain on the body by continually creating this effect. In the long run, this can lead to tiredness and ill health, which is the body's way of saying stop. Herbal teas can be a delicious and healthy substitute for caffeine drinks and can replenish our energy.

### HERBAL REMEDIES
Herbal remedies are very effective in supporting the nervous system through the use of nervine tonics such as ginseng, skullcap, oats and vervain. Nervine relaxants include camomile, crampbark, hops, hyssop, lavender, limeblossom, motherwort, passion flower, St John's wort, skullcap and valerian. Some of these help to relax the muscles and soothe the nerves, creating a feeling of ease.

### AILMENTS
Herbal treatments for the following disorders are discussed here: stress and anxiety; depression; insomnia; hyperactivity; headache; migraine; neuralgia; and nervous exhaustion.

*Talking with others who understand your problems may help to bring new solutions to traumatic and stressful situations.*

## STRESS

Stress is the body's natural reaction to any situation that places extra demands on us. It can have a positive or negative effect, depending on our response. Long-term stress, however, can put strain on the nervous system and other areas of the body that may be weak or prone to reacting to stress. Herbs can help to prevent debility and give you the energy needed to make positive choices in stressful situations. Nerve tonics, such as skullcap and vervain, taken as teas, help to strengthen the nervous system. Oats, taken daily as porridge or gruel, are an essential part of the treatment, especially if there is general debility. Vitamins C and B-Complex are also needed during stressful times.

### GINSENG
Ginseng is another important nerve tonic that is used when there are other symptoms of weakness. It is classified as an adaptogen. Adaptogens help improve the body's ability to adapt to different situations, enabling it to avoid reaching breaking-point or collapse. Take ginseng as a Chinese decoction, tincture, medicinal wine, or powder in capsules.

## ANXIETY

Anxiety can be the result of on-going stress or a traumatic event in our lives. Sometimes it can become a habitual response, even to situations where there is no cause for worry. Using herbs to help ease feelings of anxiety reminds us of the strength that comes from feeling peaceful in our daily lives. A herbal decoction of valerian,

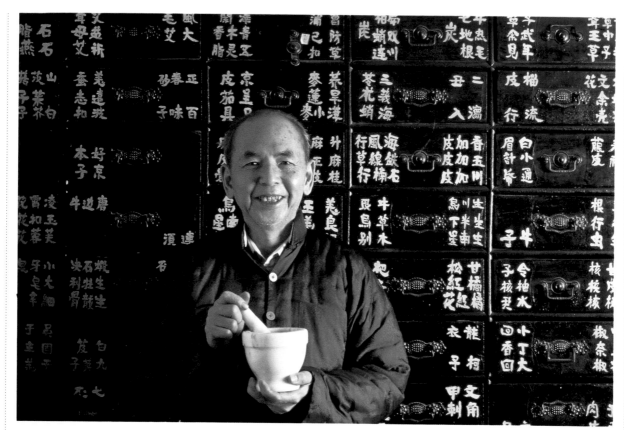

skullcap and verbena calms anxiety and builds up the nervous system. Herbal baths with lavender, rosemary or camomile help to ease tension. Drink infusions of limeblossom, camomile, passion flower, hops, hyssop or motherwort to replace caffeine drinks such as coffee and black tea.

## DEPRESSION

Depression can be the result of a long-term physical illness, general tiredness or external difficulties. Herbal treatment can help to lift depression and strengthen the body, creating a more positive attitude to cope with its other causes. If there is general debility with the depression, try a Chinese herbal decoction of ginseng (*see* p. 32). Take wild oats, skullcap, or vervain daily as teas or tinctures to help lift the spirits and replace nutrients. For depression following an illness, drink a tea made from rosemary, vervain and dandelion leaves. Ginkgo is another herbal supplement which helps to alleviate depression, especially in the elderly. Since depression can be a serious problem, professional treatment using commercially prepared standardized extracts may be necessary. In this case, be sure to consult a health professional.

## SEASONAL ADJUSTMENT DISORDER (SAD)

St John's wort will help to brighten moods, and has recently been used to treat SAD, in which depression sets in during the winter months. Add this to other herbs used for treating depression to make a medicinal tea or tincture.

*In Chinese herbal medicine, ginseng has been used for more than 2000 years as a tonic to help to strengthen the nervous system.*

## INSOMNIA

Sleepless nights can be caused by tension, anxiety, overwork, physical pain, too much caffeine and too little fresh air and exercise. Insomnia can create all sorts of other problems, such as chronic tiredness, lack of concentration and depression. A good night's rest is healing for both the body and the mind.

### HERBAL REMEDIES
A warm herbal bath before bed, using lavender, limeflower, camomile or rose will ease tense muscles and calm an overactive mind. Try drinking camomile as a tea or tincture before going to bed (*see* Herbal

Methods section). Other herbs that can be taken as infusions are lime-blossom, catnip, lemon balm or hops. Sleep-pillows of lavender, rose petals or hops can be tucked under your pillow at night. For persistent insomnia, try a combination of passion flower, valerian and hops as a tincture. Take half a teaspoonful in a small amount of water one hour before bedtime, and repeat the dose if you wake in the night.

### CHINESE REMEDIES
Chinese herbal patent formulas have several remedies useful for insomnia. *Suan Zao Ren Tang Pian* helps to treat insomnia with mental agitation, restlessness and irritability. It calms the *shen*, the spirit of the heart. *Tian Wang Bu Xin Wan* (Heavenly King Benefit Heart Pill) also calms the *shen* and helps with insomnia that may result after a long illness or with ageing. It can be used to treat insomnia and other symptoms due to a hyperactive thyroid.

**Four approaches to helping to relieve stress, tension and anxiety**

MEDICINE
*Orthodox drugs*
*Herbal medicine*
*Homeopathy*
*Diet*
*Bach Flower Remedies*

PSYCHOTHERAPY
*Counselling*
*Hypnotherapy*
*Psychiatry*
*Tender loving care*
*(TLC)*

BODY WORK
*Exercise*
*Massage*
*Yoga*
*Herbal baths*
*Aromatherapy*
*Acupuncture*
*Alexander Technique*

SPIRITUAL HEALING
*Prayer*
*Meditation*
*Music*
*Poetry*
*Gardening*
*Country walks*
*Tranquillity*

*Chinese herbs are roots, bark, leaves or berries of plants. These are combined to help balance the properties of each herb.*

# HYPERACTIVITY

Hyperactivity is a growing concern among parents. Lack of concentration, an inability to sit still, temper tantrums and sleep difficulties can all be symptoms. They will vary with each child, but hypertension often has a profound effect on both the child and the parent. A combination of good diet and herbal treatment will help with this problem.

### FOODS TO AVOID
Provide a diet that is as pure and natural as possible, avoiding artificial colourings and additives, which are now required by law to be listed on packaged foods. Notice if any foods spark off reactions in

the child, since hyperactivity can be related to food allergies. Make sure that the child has plenty of fresh air and exercise to help him or her let off steam.

### HERBAL REMEDIES

A herbal tea of red clover should be taken three times a day over a period of time to cleanse any toxicity from the body. Red clover is also a nervine relaxant. If stronger relaxants are needed, use oats and vervain as well. Oats can be given as porridge and the vervain as a tea or tincture. Relaxing herbal baths, using camomile or lavender, will help to calm the child before bed. Try a vaporizer or aromatherapy oil burner with these herbs or essential oils to create a peaceful atmosphere (*see* Herbal Methods section).

## HEADACHES

Headaches can be a symptom of an overstretched nervous system due to stress and exhaustion, but there are other causes which need to be taken into consideration. For example, they can be related to the menstrual cycle, allergies, high and low blood pressure, digestive problems, low blood sugar, eyestrain, poor posture and back problems. It is important to find out the cause, especially if the headaches are chronic.

### HERBAL PAIN RELIEF

Herbal treatment for pain relief includes many herbs which have a wide range of associated actions. Consult the Herbal Directory to find the herbs best suited for an individual. Suggestions include camomile, chrysanthemum (*ju hua*), feverfew, lavender, lemon balm, limeflower, passion flower, rosemary, skullcap, St John's wort

and valerian. Choose several herbs in combination or on their own to make an infusion or decoction (*see* Herbal Methods section), and drink as needed to ease the headache. Herbal baths using lavender, rosemary or peppermint may help lessen the pain.

### TENSION HEADACHES

Rosemary, crampbark and valerian relieve the neck and shoulder tension that sometimes accompanies headache. If stress and anxiety are involved, use infusions of vervain, camomile, skullcap and passion flower to calm and strengthen the nervous system and ease the pain. Drink as a tea when needed.

## MIGRAINES

Migraines are intense headaches often accompanied with symptoms of nausea and vomiting. Visual disturbances can be early warning signs that a

migraine may be about to begin. Dizziness and light sensitivity indicate that the best treatment is to lie down and rest in a dark room.

### COMMON CAUSES

Studies have shown that in most cases migraines can be aggravated by dietary factors, stress, hormonal imbalances, or structural problems. Allergic reactions to certain foods – most common of which are red meat, chocolate, hard cheeses, coffee and red wine – can trigger migraines. Stressful situations can also be a trigger for migraines, although many sufferers cope well while the pressure is on them and find the migraine sets in when they relax. Migraines related to hormonal imbalances will occur regularly each month with changes in the menstrual cycle. See other sections of the book to find herbal advice to strengthen the digestion, calm and relax the nerves and balance the hormones. Osteopathic or chiropractic treatment is needed

*It is important to find out the cause of headaches, especially if they are chronic.*

to check and treat any structural problems connected with the head, neck and spine.

### HERBAL TREATMENT

An invaluable herb for migraine treatment is feverfew, which must be taken daily as a tablet or tea for at least a month before its effectiveness can be seen. Passion flower, willow bark and valerian taken as a decoction or tincture at the first sign of pain may help to prevent the migraine from becoming too severe. Continue with a small dose of herbal medicine every few hours until the headache clears. To help ease digestive symptoms such as nausea and vomiting, sip cups of either peppermint, camomile or meadowsweet tea.

# NEURALGIA

Nerve pain, or neuralgia, can be an excruciating pain that follows the path of a nerve, or a more localized pain on the place the nerve reaches the skin. Sciatica and facial neuralgia are both common types of nerve pain. They can be caused by a structural problem that may need osteopathic or chiropractic treatment. Generally there is some debility, and this is why the nerve pain and inflammation does not go away. Include lots of green vegetables and fruit in your diet, with extra supplements of vitamin B-Complex for a while. Rest and relax to allow the body to heal itself.

### HERBAL TREATMENT

Herbal treatment should include infusions, decoctions or tinctures of ginseng, hops, passion flower, St John's wort and valerian. Choose the herb that suits your overall complaint, and take it three times a

*Rest is essential to relieve nervous exhaustion, which can result from long-term stress and anxiety.*

day. Lavender and St John's wort oil rubbed into the painful area, will give temporary relief. If neuralgia is associated with shingles, take a tea or tincture of echinacea and marigold for three months to cleanse and heal the body.

# NERVOUS EXHAUSTION

Long-term stress and anxiety, overwork, insomnia and poor diet may lead to low vitality and nervous exhaustion. During stressful periods, vitamins and minerals are used by the body in higher concentrations. It is often more difficult to eat well during these times. Greater amounts of tea, coffee and alcohol may be consumed, all of which further deplete the body. This may create a destructive cycle where energy is not being replenished, and there is little left to cope with the difficult situation. If nervous exhaustion reaches an extreme level, a collapse or breakdown occurs, which then forces rest and

recovery. Rest, vitamin supplements of B-Complex and C, and herbal treatment will assist the recovery of vitality.

### WESTERN HERBAL TREATMENT

Use a tea of red clover, dandelion leaves and burdock to help cleanse the body, especially if large amounts of coffee, tea and alcohol have been consumed. Nettle can help to tone and remineralize the system. Nervine tonics such as oats, vervain and skullcap will strengthen the nervous system. Drink these herbs three times a day, and avoid coffee, alcohol and tobacco. Add liquorice root to support their effect on the adrenal glands, which are often weakened by overwork and overconsumption of caffeine.

### CHINESE HERBAL TREATMENT

The Chinese herbs ginseng and astragalus will boost the physical energy as well as having a calming effect. Take either one of them as a Chinese herbal decoction twice a day.

# THE IMMUNE SYSTEM

*The immune system keeps us healthy by fighting off the many organisms that attack the body, including bacteria, viruses, fungi, parasites and allergens. It is a complex system that is well integrated into all aspects of the body and has many levels of defence.*

The body has many intricate mechanisms to fight off potentially harmful micro-organisms. Tears and saliva are antiseptic; the nose and chest have tiny hairs and sticky mucus in which to trap organisms; and the skin is coated in a protective oil. To get rid of harmful organisms, the stomach and vagina contain acids; the bladder flushes such organisms out; and the bowels contain gut flora that help to clear them. The blood contains white blood cells which attack an infection. If these natural systems fail, the lymphatic system comes into action, and antibodies are produced to fight the invading mico-organisms.

## THE ROLE OF THE LYMPHATIC SYSTEM

The lymphatic system is a network of tiny vessels which carry lymph, a colorless liquid which picks up debris and micro-organisms, and lymph nodes, which are concentrations of white blood cells. The lymph nodes are situated in groups in the neck, armpits, groin, chest, and abdomen. White blood cells consume harmful microbes and filter out debris. They also produce antibodies, which are carried through the body via the lymph. When the body is under attack, the lymph nodes swell and feel tender.

## INTERACTION WITH THE BODY

The immune system is integrated into the body as described above. A healthy diet and good digestion are important in the production of lymph. Lymph is moved through the body by the contractions of the muscles. The liver is the main detoxifying organ in the body, where the debris from infections is filtered out from the blood.

## THE CHINESE MEDICINE APPROACH

In Chinese medicine, the immune system is regarded as the *wei qi*, or defensive energy, that surrounds the body. It is closely related to the digestive system, and herbs that strengthen this, such as ginseng and astragalus (*huang qi*), help to build up this energy. If the *wei qi* is strong, infections are prevented from taking hold in the body.

## BOOSTING IMMUNITY

There are several factors that impair the immune system and weaken it. Stress, a poor diet and nutritional deficiencies, environmental pollution, injury and surgery, digestive problems and the over-use of antibiotics can all impair the immune system. A positive and relaxed state of mind will help to increase the body's ability to cope with allergies and disease. A wholefood diet, high in organic fruits and vegetables, nuts, beans and pulses, and unrefined oils will provide a good foundation for a healthy immune system. Using herbs that strengthen the immune system and help recovery from illness and injury, will enhance healthy functioning in all systems of the body.

## STRENGTHENING THE IMMUNE SYSTEM

There are many herbs that will help to boost the immune system. Garlic is one of nature's best antimicrobial products which helps to prevent infections, even in those who have become immune to antibiotics. Take one or two garlic perles morning and night. Borage has a supportive and restorative effect on the adrenal glands. It is used to help with depression and other stress-related problems, as well as to aid convalescence. Wild yam has an anti-inflammatory effect, helping to relieve symptoms of infection and allergy. It is also a tonic for the digestive tract and liver. As an alternative to antibiotics, echinacea is useful for fighting infections and cleansing the blood and lymphatic system.

## How the immune system works

*The blood capillaries are impermeable to large molecules such as proteins. Any protein which leaks into the tissue fluid from cells or plasma cannot therefore enter the bloodstream. These molecules are absorbed, along with some tissue fluid, by the lymphatic system.*

Capillary

90%

Tissue fluid

Protein 100%

10%

*Lymphatic capillaries are found in all the tissues of the body, except those of the central nervous system.*

*The capillaries unite to form lymphatic vessels, which have large numbers of valves. They all drain into lymph nodes, which filter the lymph and pass it on to further vessels.*

*Camomile and yarrow contain natural antihistamines, which help reduce inflammation in acute allergies.*

*The lymph vessels of the upper right part of the body finally drain into the right lymphatic duct, which empties the lymph into the right subclavian vein.*

*The vessels from the rest of the body join to form the thoracic duct, which empties into the left subclavian vein. The lymph in the thoracic duct contains a high proportion of fats absorbed from the villi of the small intestine.*

*Ginseng helps to increase the white blood cell count.*

*Echinacea is good at fighting infections and supporting the immune system.*

*Eating garlic regularly helps to boost immunity and prevent infections.*

*Convalescence after illness should include rest, a healthy diet and herbal treatment to help boost immunity.*

### CHINESE HERBS

Astragalus (*huang qi*) can be used to increase energy and build resistance to disease. Chinese angelica (*dang qui*) helps to restore energy and vitality, and stimulates white blood cell and antibody formation. Liquorice (*gan cao*) can be taken during recovery from illness, and helps to support the functions of the liver and adrenal glands; it also enhances the immune system by stimulating the formation of white blood cells and antibodies. Ginseng is a wonderful remedy which boosts immunity and energy and enables the body to cope with stress. It can increase the white blood cell count, and benefits the liver and spleen.

### AILMENTS

In this section, ailments related to a low-immune system will be discussed. Herbal and more conventional treatments for infections will be reviewed. Suggestions will be given on reducing the side-effects of antibiotics and other drugs. Ways of discovering and recognizing possible allergic substances, and treatment for allergies, will be given.

## INFECTIONS

Bacterial and viral infections are the most common form of acute illnesses. Bacteria can invade the respiratory and the digestive systems, causing complaints such as throat, ear and chest infections, and gastric upsets. Colds, influenza and the infectious diseases of childhood are often due to viral infections. Supplements of vitamin C can be used to boost immunity. Take up to 500 mg three or four times a day. If this is more than the body needs, it will be excreted through the urine, and may cause diarrhoea. Garlic will also fight both viral and bacterial infections.

## ANTIBIOTICS

If there is a lot of pain or a high fever, antibiotics are valuable in fighting bacterial infections, such as those of the inner ear, throat or chest. If the body temperature goes above 40°C (104°F), or there are symptoms of confusion, loss of consciousness or twitching, consult a doctor immediately. If the fever or pain lasts for more than three days without signs of improvement, professional medical advice is needed. Antibiotics can be useful for infections that are not clearing with other forms of treatment, particularly when the person is showing signs of weakening from the illness.

### DIETARY ADVICE

If antibiotics are prescribed, herbal and dietary treatments can help prevent side-effects and boost the immune system to avoid repeated attacks of infections. Side-effects include gastric upsets such as constipation, diarrhoea and abdominal pain and bloating. Garlic can be taken to boost the immune system, to protect the liver and to prevent gastric disturbances. Eat live yogurt or take lactobacillus tablets (acidophilus) to protect the intestinal bacteria and eliminate toxins and harmful organisms via the bowel. Drink a glass of water with a teaspoon of cider vinegar daily to help clear the digestive tract. Drink plenty of water and urinate frequently to flush the toxins through the system and help the kidneys and bowels with elimination.

### HELPFUL HERBS

The liver and the kidneys are involved in the filtering of toxins that are the result of drug therapy, including antibiotics. They are susceptible to stress from this process, and herbal treatment can be used to strengthen and support them. Chinese angelica, rosemary and dandelion root can support the action of the liver and help it to break down toxins. Dandelion root, milk thistle, agrimony and echinacea help to repair liver damage that may have been caused by long-term use of drugs. Celery seed will support the kidneys with the filtering and elimination of toxins. Take these herbs as teas or tinctures as needed (*see* Herbal Methods section).

# ALLERGIES

An allergic reaction is caused when the immune system reacts against a substance that is not potentially infectious or harmful, but may in fact be nutritious and beneficial. The linings of mucous membranes in the digestive and respiratory tracts become inflamed and release a chemical called histamine. This can cause inflammation of the nasal passages, overproduction of mucus, eye irritation, asthma, diarrhoea and urticaria (hives). Hayfever, asthma, eczema, bowel problems, migraines and headaches can all be symptoms of allergic reactions.

### FOOD ALLERGIES

The most common food allergies are to wheat, dairy produce, eggs, oranges, tomatoes, peanuts, gluten (a protein found in oats, wheat, barley and rye), food additives and yeast. If a food allergy is suspected, remove one of the foods from the diet for two weeks. Sometimes the symptom of the allergy disappears within a few days. At other times it can take much longer and become worse before it gets better. Introduce the food back into the diet in a small amount every few days until it can be tolerated. Some allergies are for life, for example, those related to strawberries, penicillin and shellfish. It is possible to be allergic to more than one food or additive so consult a qualified nutritionist to try out a complete food allergy elimination diet.

### HERBAL TREATMENT

Combine echinacea, red clover, borage and liquorice and drink as a tea, three times daily, over several months to help boost the immune system. A tea of marshmallow and slippery elm before meals will soothe the digestive tract if there are symptoms of upset. Camomile or yarrow teas contain natural antihistamines and help to reduce inflammations in acute allergies; they can be taken frequently. Nettle tea or soup also helps to calm allergic responses and is strengthening to the body.

### A CHINESE REMEDY

The patent remedy *Bu Zhong Yi Qi Wan* (Central Qi Pills) contains the Chinese herbs ginseng, astragalus (*huang qi*), angelica (*dang gui*), and liquorice (*gan cao*). These herbs help to boost the immune system and strengthen the body, preventing allergic reactions from having their full effect. The remedy is useful in the treatment of food allergies where symptoms affect the digestive system, combined with those of general signs of weakness, such as tiredness, a pale complexion, weak limbs and shortness of breath.

# HERBAL DIRECTORY

*From* Achillea millefolium *to* Zingiber officinale, *this section provides information on the applications, methods of preparation, dosages and contraindications of 50 common herbs.*

# YARROW
*Compositae* ACHILLEA MILLEFOLIUM

This herb is a native of Europe, naturalized in North America and grown in many other countries where there is a mild climate. The plant grows to about 1m (3 ft) and can be found in various types of terrain. The leaves are alternate, split into many fronds, and the flowers are white or pink.

### History

The name yarrow comes from the Old English *gearwe*, while the botanical name *Achillea* denotes its reputed usage by Achilles, who during the Trojan War employed it to staunch bleeding wounds on the battlefield. The name *millefolium* refers to the finely divided leaves: *mille* meaning thousand, and *folium* leaves. Its use to stem bleeding also gave it common names such as soldier's wound wort and knight's milfoil. Native Americans have long used this herb as a remedy. Vogel states that a report dated 1794 showed that yarrow was used on cuts by the Illinois and Miami tribes. The Ute name for yarrow designated it a wound medicine, and many tribes treated bruises or skin problems with it. The Micmacs used it to promote sweating in colds, and others used it for fevers.

### Parts used

Herb.

### Active constituents

Volatile oil, containing salicylic acid and sesquiterpene lactones; azulene, including chamazulene; flavonoids, including apigenin; alkaloids and plant acids.

### How it works in the body

The apigenin has been shown to have anti-inflammatory and anti-spasmodic properties, while the azulenes and salicylic acids are also both antispasmodic. The alkaloids have a hemostatic action, which confirms its usage as a remedy to stop bleeding. Chamazulene (as in camomile) is antiallergenic. This herb has an action in many different systems of the body. It is probably best known for its action in the respiratory system, its diaphoretic (increases sweating) properties being used in treating colds and fevers. It can also be used for allergy, for example, hayfever. Its combined properties make it useful as a tonic following flu or illness, to promote digestion where there is little appetite. In the cardiovascular system its antispasmodic and slightly diuretic action make it valuable for lowering high blood pressure and improving the venous circulation. In the reproductive system, it is known as a menstrual regulator, which also helps to reduce heavy bleeding. Conversely, it can also bring on a period.

### Applications

As a tea, yarrow can be taken with other herbs (*see* Herbal Methods, infusions: cold and flu tea p.17) 200 ml (8 fl oz) three times daily. As a tincture, take 1 ml (20 drops) three times a day.

### Indications

- Colds, flu, and fever.
- Allergies such as hayfever.
- As a tonic for the digestion in convalescence.
- High blood pressure.
- Varicose veins and other vascular problems.
- To regulate periods and reduce heavy periods.

### Contraindications

**Do not** use in pregnancy. Yarrow has, in rare cases, been known to cause an allergic reaction; if this occurs consult a practitioner.

# LADY'S MANTLE

*Rosaceae* ALCHEMILLA VULGARIS

Lady's mantle is a native of Britain and Europe. It grows to around 30 cm (1 ft) high. The lobed leaves are soft, downy and arranged in a rosette, from which the tiny yellow-green flowers rise on stalks.

### History

The name lady's mantle first appeared in the *History of Plants* (1532). The name derives from its association with the Virgin Mary (note that it is lady's mantle not ladies'), since the leaves are said to resemble a cape, or mantle. The scientific name *Alchemilla* comes from the Arabic for alchemy, the pseudoscientific method by which it was believed base metals could be changed into gold. In the Middle Ages the herb was used to staunch bleeding and to heal sores.

### Parts used

Leaves and flowers.

### Active constituents

Tannins, salicylic acid.

### How it works in the body

The tannins act as an astringent, helping to reduce bleeding, particularly in the reproductive system, thus making it a valuable treatment for excessive menstrual bleeding and in the menopause. It is an excellent tonic for the uterus. The herb's properties enable it to act as a hormonal balancer, which means that it also has the effect of normalizing an irregular cycle. The salicylic acid acts as a mild painkiller, helping to ease painful periods. The protective layer formed by the tannins on the tissues mean that this herb is also helpful in the digestive system where there is diarrhoea.

### Applications

Use the leaves as an infusion, 200 ml (8 fl oz), three times a day to help regularize the menstrual cycle and relieve heavy bleeding. In stomach upsets where there is diarrhoea, take the tincture, 2 ml (40 drops), three times a day.

### Indications

- Heavy menstrual or menopausal bleeding.
- To help normalize an irregular menstrual cycle.
- Cramping pains associated with a period.
- Diarrhoea in digestive disorders.

### Contraindications

Do **not** take this herb during pregnancy.

---

**Benefits of lady's mantle**

Gently astringent in gastric upsets

Useful in menopause

Eases period pains and cramps

Helps balance irregular menstrual cycle

# GARLIC
*Liliaceae* ALLIUM SATIVUM

This plant is a member of the onion family, and is cultivated all over the world for use in cooking, as well as for its medicinal properties. The leaves are long and narrow, but the part that is used, the bulb, is divided into cloves enveloped in a paper-like skin.

### History

Garlic is well known throughout many cultures and countries. The Greeks, Romans and Egyptians all valued its magical as well as edible properties. The name garlic comes from the Old English *gar,* meaning spear, and *leac,* meaning leek, a reference to the shape of the leaves. In England, its antiseptic properties were recognized early and it was the main ingredient in 'four thieves vinegar', used as protection against the plague by thieves who robbed the bodies of victims. During the First World War, garlic was used to prevent sepsis of wounds. Chicago derived its name from a Native American name for wild garlic, and its use in North America is of long-standing: the Cheyenne used one variety as a poultice for treating boils, and in Pennsylvania in the 18th century, garlic and onions were given to children with croup

### Parts used

Bulb only.

### Active constituents

Volatile oil, including allicin, enzymes, vitamins A, B, and C and flavonoids.

### How it works in the body

The volatile oil, which produces garlic's distinctive odour, contains allicin, which has been proved to have an antibiotic effect on *staphylococcus aureus,* among other bacterial infections, and it is effective against *candida albicans.* The allicin has, in addition, a hypoglycemic effect, reducing blood sugar levels. Further, it has shown an antithrombotic action, reducing blood clotting, and lowering blood pressure and reducing cholesterol.

### Applications

Use peeled, crushed cloves of fresh garlic in vinegar to dress salads, and add garlic cloves to cooking to benefit the immune system as a whole. Garlic syrup can be used to counter sore throats and coughs; take 5 ml (1 tsp) four or five times a day. Garlic is obtainable commercially as a juice and also as tablets and capsules (perles).

### Indications

- Chest infections, including bronchitic ailments.
- Coughs, colds and flu.
- To reduce catarrh.
- To reduce cholesterol, lower blood pressure and prevent the clotting of blood in thrombosis.
- Digestive problems.
- To reduce blood sugar levels in late-onset diabetes.

### Contraindications

Do not give raw garlic medicinally to children under the age of 12 without the supervision of a herbal or medical practitioner. Although some people do eat garlic raw, it is advisable to eat it only with other foods, since it is very strong and can cause griping pains if consumed on its own. Garlic may be taken alongside conventional antibiotics and diabetic medication, but conventional medicines must not be discontinued without advice from a medical or herbal practitioner, since this can be dangerous.

# ALOE VERA

*Liliaceae* ALOE VERA

A succulent with long, fleshy leaves, aloe vera comes originally from Africa but is now cultivated all over the world. It is often seen as a house plant.

### History

Aloe vera has been used for thousands of years. Some of its most famous users are said to include Alexander the Great and Cleopatra. Commercially, it is added to many skin-care products.

### Parts used

The leaves contain two different liquids, both of which can be used medicinally. The first is a clear gel, obtained by breaking the upper parts of the leaves, which is used externally as a healing agent for cuts, scrapes, and burns. The second is a bitter yellow substance, 'bitter aloes' which is derived from the rind of the plant. This liquid is very strong and acts as a laxative when taken internally. The 'bitters' should never be allowed to come into contact with the skin, and they should only be employed as a laxative under the supervision of a practitioner.

### Active constituents

Polysaccharides, the gel, contains anthraquinone glycosides, known as Aloin, and aloe-emodin, glyco-proteins, saponins and resins.

### How it works in the body

The properties of aloe vera mean that it is excellent as a vulnary, or wound healer, mainly due to the anthraquinones, and the gel is particularly noted for its soothing quality when used on the skin. The gel is also useful internally as a healer, particularly in the digestive system. In general, the gel is good for the immune system. The laxative effect derives from the irritant nature of the yellow sap, which in lower doses stimulates the colon producing a bowel movement. However, in larger doses it acts as a purgative, giving a much more vigorous action, which can result in griping pains. New scientific interest is in the use of aloe vera for the treatment of radiation burns.

### Application

The upper, fleshy part of the leaves is broken off and split apart to obtain the clear gel. This can be applied directly to the skin twice a day.

### Indications

- Aloe vera can be used as a first-aid remedy, to help heal cuts, scrapes and grazes. It is also useful for mild burns.
- To soothe itchy or dry skin.
- To help with digestive tract problems such as ulcers.

### Contraindications

This herb stimulates the uterus, so it should **never** be used during pregnancy or while breastfeeding. It should also should be avoided by those suffering from kidney disease.

### Benefits of aloe vera

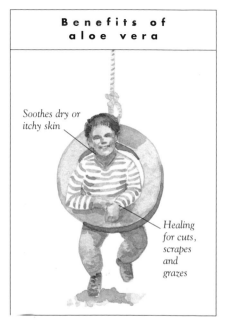

Soothes dry or itchy skin

Healing for cuts, scrapes and grazes

# MARSHMALLOW

*Malvaceae* ALTHAEA OFFICINALIS

This plant is native to Europe and Britain and is naturalized in North America. It grows to about 2m (6 ft), and has pale green oval leaves covered in soft down, and pinkish white flowers. The root is white. It is found in damp, marshy locations, by rivers and close to the seaside.

### History

The family name *Malvaceae* comes from *malake*, soft, and *Althaea* is from the Greek *althein*, to heal. This plant was used by the Romans and Egyptians as a food of great delicacy, and the roots have long been boiled and eaten as a vegetable in poorer regions. Its medicinal value has a long history: Arabic physicians used the leaves as a poultice for inflammation, and the Roman historian Pliny said, 'Whosoever shall take a spoonful of the Mallows shall that day be free from all diseases that may come to him.' The confectionery known as marshmallow contains no trace of the plant, but the name has persisted due to the mucilaginous quality of the main constituents. In France, the flowers are one of the main ingredients of a cold remedy known as *tisane de quatre fleurs*.

### Parts used
Leaves, flowers and roots.

### Active constituents
Root: mucilage 18–35 per cent, including polysaccharides, pectin, asparagine and tannins. Leaves: mucilage, flavonoids, coumarins and polyphenolic acids.

### How it works in the body
The main ingredient is the mucilage, which acts to soothe and protect tissues in the body. Long used for complaints of the respiratory system, marshmallow is useful where inflammation occurs in bronchitis and pleurisy and where there is a dry cough. It is also useful in the digestive system to help heal ulcers and the gastric inflammation generally occurring in conditions such as irritable bowel syndrome. Mallow is also used to calm irritated tissues in urinary tract infections such as cystitis. In skin problems where there are ulcers or boils, it is soothing and healing, and can be used as a poultice.

### Applications
For digestive disorders, respiratory complaints, and urinary tract infections, the flowers may be used as an infusion; take 200 ml (8 fl oz), three times daily. Use also as a tincture, 2 ml (40 drops), three times daily. Prepare as a poultice for boils or ulcerations and as a drawing paste or cream for stings, splinters, and boils. Externally, use the infusion as a wash for irritated skin.

### Indications
- Respiratory complaints, bronchitic complaints, and dry coughs.
- Digestion, including irritable bowel syndrome, diverticulitis, ulcers and excess stomach acid.
- Urinary tract infections.
- Topically, as a wash for skin conditions.
- As a poultice for boils and ulcers.
- As a drawing paste for stings and boils.

# CHINESE ANGELICA

*Umbelliferae* ANGELICA SINENSIS *(∂ang gui)*

There are three main types of angelica: European, Chinese, and American. All three are helpful for the digestion and the circulation, but there are some specific differences in how they function, so they cannot be used interchangeably. The variety described here has been selected for its wide-ranging applications.

### History

Chinese angelica strongly resembles its Western counterpart, but its application differs in certain respects. While being used for the circulation, it is mainly used for women's conditions, and its use is increasingly respected.

### Parts used

Roots, rhizomes, leaves, stalks and seeds.

### Active constituents

Volatile oil, coumarins, vitamin B12.

### How it works in the body

Chinese angelica's constituents make it especially valuable for treating women's reproductive problems. Its combined action as a circulatory and blood tonic means it is useful during the menopause for symptoms including aches and pains, as well as helping with irregular and absent periods. Its antispasmodic actions also help with painful periods. In China it is used to nourish the blood and prevent anaemia, blurred vision, tinnitus and palpitations. Like garden angelica, it is a warming, carminative herb for the digestion and has been found to help where there is long-term liver damage or infection. It is used in cases of constipation. The rhizome has an antibiotic quality, which is helpful in cases where there are sores and abscesses. The Chinese properties are sweet, acrid, bitter and warm.

### Applications

The root is added to foods in China as a tonic for the circulation. It is excellent with other herbs as a wine; take a wineglassful a day. As an infusion, take one or two cups daily. Chinese dosage is 3–15 g (⅛–¾ oz).

### Indications

- Painful or irregular periods.
- Menopause, as a tonic for the reproductive system.
- As a circulatory herb for cold hands and feet.
- Improves digestion.
- Impaired liver function.

### Contraindications

**Do not** take during pregnancy.

# BURDOCK

*Compositae* ARCTIUM LAPPA (*niu bang zi*)

Chinese pharmaceutical name: *fructus arctii lappae*

Of European origin, this plant has also established itself in China and the United States. Burdock belongs to the thistle family and has large, broad leaves and purple flowers with tiny hooks.

### History

The botanical name is thought to be derived from the Greek *arktos*, meaning bear (an allusion to its rough texture) and *lappa*, meaning to take hold of. The name burdock combines bur, a seedhead with hooks, and dock, a reference to the large leaves. It forms the basis of the cleansing drink known as dandelion and burdock. According to Vogel, an American doctor, many Native Americans used this herb – the Plains Indians for ceremonial purposes and the Potawatomis as a tea and general tonic and blood purifier. In Japan, its roots are eaten for their fibre, which in tests on animals has been shown to protect the liver from the effects of food colourants.

### Parts used

Roots and leaves.

### Active constituents

Lignans, amino acids and polyacetylenes in the roots. In the leaves, sesquiterpenes, bitter glycosides, arctigenin, inulin, organic acids and oils.

### How it works in the body

The plant's diuretic effect has made it a traditional remedy for gout and kidney stones. It has also been used in rheumatic conditions. Its main value is as an alterative or blood cleanser to remove waste products from the body, and it is employed to treat conditions such as psoriasis, eczema, boils, and other skin complaints. It lowers blood sugar levels, and the arctigenin has been shown to be effective against tumors. The fresh root is thought to have an antibiotic quality, probably due to the polyacetylenes. In China, it is used for catarrhal conditions and when there is a fever, cough and sore throat, and in infective diseases such as mumps and the early stages of measles. Burdock also stimulates the digestion and aids the liver, and in China is a remedy for constipation. The Chinese properties are acrid, bitter and cold.

### Applications

The roots are prepared as a decoction for skin problems; half a cup should be taken once a day. The tincture should be taken only for short periods, 1 ml (20 drops), twice a day for up to four weeks. Burdock is best used in the traditional manner, in combination with a liver herb such as dandelion. Externally, use the leaves either as a poultice for boils, or as an ointment for dry skin. As a hair rinse, the decoction is thought to help with alopecia, or hair loss. The Chinese dosage is 3–9 g (⅛–½ oz).

### Indications

- For its antibiotic properties in infectious illnesses to speed recovery.
- Internally for skin complaints, including eczema, psoriasis, acne and boils.
- Externally as a poultice for boils and abscesses.
- Arthritic conditions.
- In small amounts to promote digestion and encourage the appetite.

### Contraindications

**Do not** use in pregnancy.

# MUGWORT
*Compositae* ARTEMISIA VULGARIS *(moxa-ai ye)*
Chinese pharmaceutical name: *folium artemisiae argyi*

This herb of European origin is also found in China. The plant, which often occurs on wasteground, grows to about 1 m (3 ft) and can be very straggly, depending on soil conditions. The deeply lobed, smooth leaves are green on top and downy white underneath, and the reddish yellow flowers grow in spikes.

### History
Mugwort is said to have acquired its common name from being used as an ingredient of beers before hops began to be used, the mug being the vessel or drinking cup. Another suggestion is that the name comes from a word for moths, since it has a reputation for keeping these insects at bay. In the Middle Ages it was believed that John the Baptist wore a girdle made from the herb, and one of its names is St John's plant; from this it probably derived the reputation of protecting travellers, especially from evil influences. In China, it is the basis of *moxa*, a substance made into sticks, which when burnt enhances the effects of acupuncture. Culpeper recommended it ' . . . for all disorders of the stomach', it 'prevents sickness after meals and creates an appetite, but if made too strong, it disgusts the taste.'

### Parts used
Leaves.

### Active constituents
Volatile oil, vulgarin (a sesquiterpene lactone), flavonoids, coumarin derivatives, triterpenes.

### How it works in the body
Mugwort has been a traditional remedy for worms and, taken in low dosage over a period of time, can certainly help in this respect. Other functions in the digestive system include its action as a bitter, to increase appetite and promote digestion. In the reproductive system, it brings on the onset of menstruation. In Chinese herbalism, the reproductive system is again the main focus for this herb. It is used to warm the womb and stop bleeding where the menstrual cycle is prolonged, and also for uterine bleeding due to cold from deficiency. It is also used in threatened miscarriage, but this should be only under the supervision of a qualified medical or herbal practitioner. It is also used for infertility due to a cold womb and for menstrual pain. Externally it can be applied in the form of a *moxa* stick on specific acupuncture points, to help turn breech babies in the womb. The Chinese properties are bitter, acrid and warm.

### Applications
Use the tincture, 1–2 ml (20–40 drops), twice daily; as an infusion, take 100 ml (4 fl oz) twice daily. In Chinese medicine the dosage is 3–9 g (⅛–½ oz).

### Indications
- Delayed or irregular periods.
- Loss of appetite, for instance, following illness.
- Sluggish digestion, especially where there is poor absorption.
- Externally, to increase bloodflow to injured muscles, thus aiding the healing of strains and sprains.

### Contraindications
**Do not** use this herb in pregnancy. **Do not** exceed the dosage. Chinese cautions indicate it should **not** be used in cases of heat in the blood.

# ASTRAGALUS

*Leguminosae* ASTRAGALUS MEMBRANACEUS (*huang qi*)

Astragalus is a native of China, and while the herb is not so well known in the West its use is spreading. It is found in sandy areas where there is plenty of sun and grows to about 40 cm (16 in) high. The stems are hairy with up to 14 leaves growing in pairs along them.

### History

*Astragalus membranaceus* should not be confused with the American species *Astragalus nitidus*, or milk vetch, which was reportedly used by the Cheyennes as a remedy for ivy poisoning.

### Parts used

Root.

### Active constituents

Asparagine, calcyosin, formono-netin, astragalosides, kumatakenin, sterols.

### How it works in the body

One of astragalus's main properties is that of a stimulant to the immune system. American and Chinese research has confirmed its use as an energy restorative for conditions with long-term debility as a feature. It is helpful in improving resistance to colds and flu and has a similar energizing effect to that of ginseng. It has been shown that cancer patients given astragalus are better able to withstand the side-effects of orthodox treatments and have improved recovery times. Another of its main functions is that of a diuretic, which means that it is very active in the urinary tract, but it also plays a major role in the cardiovascular system, as diuretics are used to lower blood pressure. It will also help in conditions where there is water retention or oedema (swelling of the tissues due to excess water). It can be used with other herbs in cases of anaemia. In the reproductive system, astragalus is used where there is excessive bleeding, for example, during the menstrual cycle and also after childbirth due to *qi* (energy) and blood deficiency. In addition, it is beneficial in cases of prolapse of the uterus and other organs. It is valuable externally as a wound healer, especially where there is ulceration or infection leading to discharge. It can be used in the digestive system for poor appetite and digestive weakness. The Chinese properties are sweet and slightly warm.

### Applications

As a decoction, one cup of astragalus may be taken twice daily. As a tincture, take 2 ml (40 drops) three times a day. The Chinese dosage is 9–30 g (½–1½ oz).

### Indications

- As a diuretic to relieve water retention and reduce blood pressure.
- For colds and flu.
- When undergoing radiotherapy or chemotherapy, to reduce symptoms and enhance recovery.
- Excessive menstrual bleeding and after childbirth to reduce blood loss.
- Prolapse of the uterus and stomach.
- Ulcerative conditions and boils.
- Poor appetite and digestive weakness.

### Contraindications

In Western herbalism, it should **not** be taken internally for disorders of the skin. In Chinese herbalism, this herb should **not** be used for skin conditions in their early stages, or where there is heat indicated by redness. It should **not** be taken where there is food stagnation, but only where there are signs of digestive weakness.

# MARIGOLD
*Compositae* CALENDULA OFFICINALIS

Commonly known as pot marigold, this garden plant grows to about 60 cm (2 ft). It has dark green leaves and the flower resembles a large yellow or orange daisy. It is native to Europe, but is cultivated in many other countries.

### History
Its botanical name is associated with *kalendae*, or calends, the first day of the month in the Roman calendar, perhaps because of its use in treating mentrual disorders. It was later associated with the Virgin Mary and, in England, in the 17th century with Queen Mary. Its use as a culinary herb and as a medicinal plant is well documented.

### Parts used
Petals and flowerheads.

### Active constituents
Triterpenes, including calendulosides, flavonoids, volatile oil and chlorogenic acid.

### How it works in the body
One of calendula's main properties is that of an antiseptic. This makes it especially valuable externally as a healer, for cuts, scrapes and wounds. Internally, it is beneficial to many skin disorders such as acne, eczema, and psoriasis. It has a well-known antifungal action, so it is also helpful for conditions such as athlete's foot and internally for fungal-related problems such as *candida* (thrush) and diaper rash. In the cardiovascular system, it is employed both internally and externally for conditions such as varicose veins. In the digestive system, it helps with ulcerative conditions and digestive complaints and acts as a liver tonic. In the reproductive system, calendula relieves menstrual symptoms. It is also antibacterial and antiviral.

### Applications
As an infusion, take 200 ml (8 fl oz), three times daily for digestive, fungal, skin, reproductive and cardio-vascular problems. Use the infusion as a wash for varicose veins and to clean cuts and scrapes. The tincture is taken internally, 2 ml (40 drops), twice a day. As a cream, use on skin complaints such as eczema, and as an ointment on cuts and wounds, diaper rash and athlete's foot. As an infused oil, apply to the skin where there are large areas of inflammation.

### Indications
- Wound healer for cuts, scrapes and wounds.
- Acne, eczema, psoriasis and other inflammatory skin complaints.
- Diaper rash, sore and cracked nipples.
- Varicose veins.
- Fungal disorders, including *candida*.
- Stomach complaints, such as ulcers and gastric inflammation.
- Regulates the menstrual cycle and lessens a heavy flow.

### Benefits of marigold

For eczema and psoriasis

Excellent liver tonic

Antiseptic for cuts and scrapes

As an ointment for diaper rash

Anti-fungal for athlete's foot

# CAMOMILE

*Compositae* CHAMAEMELUM NOBILE/CHAMOMILLA RECUTITA

Two types of camomile, with broadly similar actions, are used medicinally. These are Roman, or garden, camomile (*Chamaemelum nobile*), and German, or wild, camomile (*Chamomilla recutita*). Both varieties grow throughout Europe.

### History

Camomile was used by the Egyptians and Romans and dedicated to their gods. The name derives from the Greek *khamaimelon*, meaning literally earthapple; indeed, the scent is faintly like that of apples. In England in the Middle Ages camomile was planted alongside walkways, since its relaxing fragrance is released when it is bruised. Often it was grown over low walls for the refreshment of the spirit. The taste of Roman camomile is, however, rather bitter when compared with that of the German species. Camomile was included among herbs taken to the New World by the Pilgrim Fathers, and in 1665 it was included in a list of medicines used by an order of nuns in Quebec in their hospital pharmacy.

### Parts used

Flowers and essential oil.

### Active constituents

Volatile oil, mainly chamazulene, flavonoids, sesquiterpene lactones, coumarins and phenolic acids.

### How it works in the body

Known as the 'mother of the gut', camomile's combined properties act as a muscle relaxant in the gut, calming and dispelling nausea and indigestion, and as a sedative for the nervous system. Externally, it can be used as an emollient cream or ointment for skin problems. It also has an antiallergenic quality.

### Applications

As an infusion, camomile may be used by children and adults (*see* guidelines for dosages p.16). Care must be taken, since the volatile oil is given off in the steam, so it is important to cover the tea while it is infusing to retain the medicinal benefits. It can also be added to the bath as in infusion, to relax and calm both children and adults. As an inhalation, it is useful for catarrh. As a cream or ointment, apply it externally once or twice daily. Use as a poultice for slow-healing wounds, and as an eyewash to relieve tired eyes. The tincture may be taken internally – up to 5 ml (1 tsp) three times a day, as required, or 5 ml (1 tsp) at night to aid sleep. The essential oil should be used externally only in a base oil for massage, or in a diffuser.

### Indications

- Indigestion, wind, excess acid and stomach ulcers. Also in nausea, especially during pregnancy, and for travel sickness, together with ginger.
- As an aid to restful sleep and to relieve stress and tension. Good for headaches.
- Respiratory complaints, such as catarrh.
- Allergic conditions such as eczema, asthma and hayfever.
- Topically, to soothe dry and itching skin.
- For tired eyes, use as an eyewash.

### Contraindications

**Do not** use the essential oil internally or externally during pregnancy.

# CHRYSANTHEMUM

*Compositae* CHRYSANTHEMUM MORIFOLIUM *(ju hua)*

Chinese pharmaceutical name: *flos chrysanthemi morifolii*

This plant grows to just over 1.5m (5 ft) high and is known in the West as florist's chrysanthemum, since it is popularly used for flower displays. It is native to China, although it is cultivated widely in the West.

### History

There are different varieties of this chrysanthemum, the white (*bai ju hua*) is used mainly as a liver herb, and is sometimes known as sweet chrysanthemum, while the yellow (*huang ju hua*) has been used to treat headaches and eye problems. It first appeared as a medicinal herb in the *Divine Husbandman's Classic of the Materia Medica* in China in AD 1.

### Parts used

Flowering tops.

### Active constituents

Alkaloids, volatile oil, sesquiterpene lactones, flavonoids, adenine, choline, stachydrine, chrysanthemin and vitamin B1.

### How it works in the body

Research has shown that chrysanthemum has an antibiotic principle that is effective in laboratory conditions against both *staphylococcus* and *streptococcus* bacteria, and so it is a valuable remedy against general infection in the body. In addition, the action of yellow chrysanthemum on headache and eye problems has been supported by research into high blood pressure. In one study, 46 patients with essential hypertension and/or atherosclerosis showed improvement in conditions ranging from headache and dizziness to insomnia after one week's treatment. The blood pressure of 35 subjects returned to normal, and continuing improvements were shown in the remainder of the patients. This herb is also used in the respiratory system to clear fever and headaches associated with colds and flu. It has long been helpful as a tonic for the eyes, especially where they are red, painful and dry, or where there is excessive watering. It is used also for spots in front of the eyes, blurred vision or dizziness. The Chinese properties are sweet, bitter and slightly cold.

### Applications

This herb may be drunk as an infusion, 200 ml (8 fl oz), three times a day. The Chinese dosage is 4.5–15 g (¼–¾ oz).

### Indications

- General conditions of infection.
- High blood pressure and related symptoms.
- Colds and flu accompanied by fever and headaches.
- As an eye tonic.

### Contraindications

The Chinese caution recommends taking care when treating patients with *qi* (energy) deficiencies or weakness, who have poor appetite and/or diarrhoea.

# BLACK COHOSH

*Ranunculaceae* CIMICIFUGA RACEMOSA

There are two types of cohosh, both originating in North America. Their families and applications are, however, quite different. Here, we focus on black cohosh, a native American herb traditionally used for women's complaints. It grows in Canada, the United States, and Europe. It has white flowers with toothed leaves and is noted for its black root. Some related species are found in China.

### History

Widely used by Native Americans, the plant was introduced into Europe. According to Vogel, Native Americans used it for reproductive disorders, debility, to promote perspiration and as a gargle for sore throats.

### Parts used

Roots and rhizome.

### Active constituents

Triterpene glycosides, isoflavones, isoferulic acid, volatile oil and tannins.

### How it works in the body

In North America, it is thought that the herb assists gynaeco-logically, helping to balance oestrogen by stabilizing it. In European herbalism, it is thought to have an oestrogenic action that actively works to reduce progesterone and promote oestrogen levels in the body. It is, therefore, used where there is a lack of oestrogen and an excess of progesterone. In the musculoskeletal system it is used as an anti-inflammatory in arthritic conditions. Its sedative qualities have applications in other systems, for example, in lowering blood pressure; in reducing spasm and tension; and in the respiratory system.

### Applications

This remedy is quite strong, and care must be taken not to exceed the stated limits. As a decoction the root should be taken only in half-cupfuls, 100 ml (4 fl oz), twice a day. The tincture may be taken, 1 ml (20 drops), three times a day.

### Indications

- Period pains and cramp.
- Gynaecological conditions where there is a lack of estrogen or an excess of progesterone.
- High blood pressure.
- Menopausal symptoms.
- Rheumatic complaints.
- Respiratory complaints such as asthma, bronchitis and whooping cough.

### Contraindications

**Do not** take during pregnancy or while breastfeeding. **Do not** use where there is low blood pressure.

### Benefits of black cohosh

In menopause for hot flushes and depression

Helps lower blood pressure

Anti-inflammatory for arthritic conditions

Eases period pains and cramps

# HAWTHORN

*Rosaceae* CRATAEGUS MONOGYNA/CRATAEGUS OXYCANTHOIDES
*(shan zha)* Chinese pharmaceutical name: *fructus crataegi*

The development of hawthorn depends on growing conditions: in hedgerows it forms a bush but can grow to a tree 9 m (30 ft) high in the open. It is found in Europe, Africa and Asia. The leaves are deeply lobed, and in the autumn the white summer flowers give way to bright red berries that contain either one seed (*monogyna*) or two seeds (*oxycanthoides*).

### History

The tree is regarded as sacred in the Christian tradition, since it is said to have formed the crown of thorns worn by Christ. Henry VII used it as a symbol of power after finding a badge from Richard III's helmet hanging on it after Richard's defeat at Bosworth Field The name *Crataegus oxycanthoides* is derived from the Greek *kratos,* meaning hard, *oxus,* sharp, and *akantha,* thorn. The common name, hawthorn, comes from the Old English *haga,* meaning a hedge. It is said that the mealy fruit was added to bread in England during the First World War, and that this helped to bring down the blood pressure of the population as a whole. Traditionally, hawthorn has been known to herbalists as the 'mother of the heart'. The Native American tribe Flambeau Ojibwas reportedly used the berries and bark for 'women's medicine'.

### Parts used

Flowers, leaves, and berries.

### Active constituents

Amines (flowers only), flavonoids, phenolic acids, tannins and ascorbic acid.

### How it works in the body

Hawthorn acts on the cardio-vascular system, regulating the heartbeat, relaxing the arteries and normalizing blood pressure, by lowering high blood pressure and raising low blood pressure. It can be used in angina and coronary artery disease to improve the bloodflow to the heart muscles. These medicinal benefits are thought to be due to a combination of the amines and the flavonoids. The effects are not instant, but taken over a period of months hawthorn will reduce symptoms and act as a tonic to the heart. In the digestive system, Chinese usage suggests that haw-thorn be given to ease digestion of meat and greasy foods, and where there is pain, distension and diarrhoea. Chinese properties are sour, sweet and slightly warm.

### Applications

An infusion of the flowers, leaves, or berries may be taken, 200 ml (8 fl oz), three times a day on a long-term basis. The tincture may be taken, 2–3 ml (40–60 drops), twice a day. There are no adverse effects from long-term use, and discontinuing use will produce no ill-effects. In Chinese medicine the dosage is 9–15 g (½–¾ oz).

### Indications

- Symptoms of angina.
- Low or high blood pressure, to restore to normal levels.
- Normalize an irregular heartbeat.
- Congestive heart failure and cardiomyopathy.

### Contraindications

**Do not** discontinue or reduce orthodox medication for any cardio-vascular condition without professional supervision. If you are receiving such medication, you must consult an orthodox or herbal practitioner before using hawthorn. Chinese cautions indicate avoidance in cases of acid regurgitation.

# PURPLE CONE FLOWER

*Compositae* ECHINACEA PURPUREA/ANGUSTIFOLIA

This plant is native to North America but, as its properties become recognized, its cultivation is becoming widespread in Europe and elsewhere in the world. The common name of this distinctive herb refers to the flower, which is shaped like a daisy, with a ring of purple florets around a central cone. The leaves are coarse and hairy.

### History

The scientific name derives from the Greek *ekhinos*, hedgehog, and refers to the prickly-looking central cone, which does resemble that animal. The herb has also been called 'snake bite' by Native Americans, who have used it for its ability to counter infection and also bites from snakes and rabid animals. This information was passed to the early settlers in North America, who continued to use it in similar circumstances. Current research has confirmed its ability to fight against infection through its antibacterial action, and has explored its role in improving and healing the immune system, especially where viral illnesses have taken hold, for example, in cases of chronic fatigue syndrome and AIDS. According to Vogel,

*Echinacea* was burned by some Native Americans as a treatment for headaches and was also used as a remedy for toothache.

### Parts used
Root, rhizome.

### Active constituents
Echinacoside (only in *purpurea*), isobutyl amides (including echinacin), polysaccharides, polyacetylenes, essential oil, alkaloids and flavonoids.

### How it works in the body
The research into how *Echinacea* works on the immune system is continuing, but it is clear that the polysaccharides play a key role in preventing viruses from taking hold in the body's cells. In particular, the herb stimulates the white T-cells within the immune system that fight off infection and keep the body healthy. Of the other constituents, the alkaloids perform an antibacterial function, and are also active against fungal infection. *Echinacea* is also used as an alterative, or blood cleanser, for the skin, helping to clear boils and other skin complaints.

### Applications
The herb is used mainly as a decoction of the root. For infections, both viral and bacterial, take 200 ml (8 fl oz), twice a day. As a tincture, take 2½ ml (50 drops/ ½ tsp), three times a day. For sore throats and mouth ulcers, combine 2 ml (40 drops) of the tincture with 2 ml (40 drops) marigold tincture and 2 ml (40 drops) myrrh tincture in 100 ml (4 fl oz) water, and gargle three times a day.

### Indications
- Colds, flu, sore throats.
- Chronic fatigue syndrome.
- HIV and AIDS.
- Bacterial infections.
- Fungal infections such as *candida* (thrush).
- Skin complaints, including boils, acne and eczema.
- Allergic conditions.

### Contraindications
In order to get the best effect from its properties, it has been suggested that in cases of HIV and AIDS it is better to take *Echinacea* for only three months at a time, and to alternate this with other immune system herbal remedies for about the same period.

# GINSENG

*Araliaceae* ELEUTHEROCOCCUS SENTICOSUS *(ren shen)*

Chinese pharmaceutical name: *radix ginseng*

There are three main types of ginseng – Siberian, panax, and American – which all belong to the same botanical family. The medicinal benefits are similar, but all three are looked at here. A native of Russia, China, Korea and Japan, the ginseng bush grows to approximately 3m (9 ft) high. The American ginseng is native to North America and the Himalayas.

### History

Russian research on Siberian ginseng has shown that its properties increase stamina and resistance to flus and other viruses. Panax ginseng has been used to improve athletic performance, and is given to improve virility in men.

### Parts used

Root.

### Active constituents

Siberian ginseng contains saponins, including eleutherosides A–F, glycans, volatile oil and two acetylenic compounds. Panax ginseng has saponin glycosides. American ginseng includes steroidal saponins.

### How it works in the body

Siberian ginseng, more stimulating to the body than panax ginseng, helps increase stamina, especially under stress. It supports the adrenal glands, which produce hormones that are responsible for repair and growth. American ginseng is very similar to panax ginseng, but milder. In Chinese terms, panax ginseng is particularly indicated for shock where there is collapse of the *qi*, or energy. It is also used for shock where there is loss of blood. In lung conditions it is used for wheezing and shortness of breath in exertion brought on by lung *qi* deficiency. It is used to treat lethargy, lack of appetite, chest and abdominal distension, chronic diarrhoea and, in severe cases, prolapse of the stomach, uterus or rectum. It benefits the heart *qi*, calms the spirit and helps palpitations with anxiety, insomnia, forgetfulness and restlessness.

### Applications

Make a decoction of the root and take 100 ml (4 fl oz), twice a day. The tincture may be taken, 2 ml (40 drops), three times a day. Tablets are available commercially; follow the instructions given. The Chinese dosage is 1–9 g (¹⁄₁₆–½ oz). Because of its cost, the herb is usually decocted separately in small amounts of water in a double boiler. (*See* Chinese herbal decoctions, p.32.)

### Indications

- Flus, colds, viral illnesses.
- Emotional and physical stress.
- Panax ginseng for male fertility problems.

### Contraindications

**Do not** take for longer than four weeks at any one time. Ginseng should not be taken by those who are fit and healthy. Do not combine with other energy stimulants, such as coffee or guarana, since this will over-stress the system. Over-use of this herb may cause headaches; stick to the recommended dosage. **Do not** take during pregnancy or while breastfeeding. **Do not** give to children under the age of 12. Chinese cautions indicate it should not be taken in cases of high blood pressure. It should be used only when there are signs of weakness. Over-dosage may cause insomnia and palpitations. The traditional antidote is mung bean soup.

# EYEBRIGHT

*Scrophulariaceae* EUPHRASIA OFFICINALIS

Eyebright is one of a family of *Euphrasias* found in Europe, Asia and North America. It is usually found on dry, chalky ground, but on rich soil can grow to about 25 cm (10 in) high. It is a semiparasite, dependent on the roots of grass, from which it draws nutrients without damaging the grass. The leaves are oval, and the flowers, which appear in summer, are white or lilac, shot through with purple veins.

### History

The botanical name *Euphrasia* is Greek for gladness – the gladness associated with the happiness of the person whose eyesight is benefited by the plant. Another tradition is that *Euphrasia* is the name given to the linnet, which used the leaves to clear the sight of her young. She gave the knowledge to humans, who named the plant in her honor. However, there is no mention of its use, before the 14th century, but in Queen Elizabeth I's time, it was used as an ale and in the 17th century wine was made from it.

### Parts used

Whole herb.

### Active constituents

Iridoid glycosides, tannins, phenolic acids, volatile oils, alkaloids, sterols.

### How it works in the body

The astringent qualities found in eyebright form a protective layer on the mucous membranes of the eyes and so reduce inflammation. This is especially beneficial for infections such as conjunctivitis. In addition, it is helpful where there is an allergic condition, such as the streaming or irritated eyes that occur with hayfever or the effects of pollution.

### Applications

As an infusion, eyebright tea may be taken internally three times a day to counter infection or allergic conditions, especially where there is watering of the eyes. Externally, it may be used either as a compress or an eyewash for sore or irritated eyes; the eyewash should not be used more than twice a day. Carefully follow the instructions in the Herbal Methods section (*see* p.22) for preparations concerning the eyes.

### Indications

- Infections or inflammations of the eye such as conjunctivitis and blephiritis.
- Allergic conditions, including hayfever and allergic rhinitis.
- Tired or reddened eyes due to overwork, pollution and tiredness.

### Contraindications

For any eye condition that does not resolve in three to four days, seek further advice from a qualified herbal or medical practitioner. For any sudden pain in the eyes or loss of vision, seek medical help immediately.

---

### Benefits of eyebright

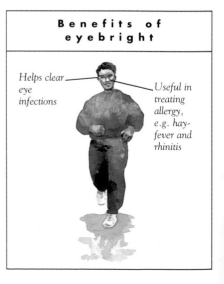

Helps clear eye infections

Useful in treating allergy, e.g. hayfever and rhinitis

# MEADOWSWEET

*Rosaceae* FILIPENDULA ULMARIA

Native to Europe, Britain and parts of Asia, this meadow plant is also naturalized in North America. It prefers damp conditions and is often found alongside riverbanks, where it can reach about 1.5 m (5 ft). The paired and toothed leaves are green on top and pale underneath. Meadowsweet blooms from June to September, and the clusters of creamy white flowers have a delicious, almondlike scent.

### History

The word *ulmaria* in its botanical name refers to the leaves, which resemble those of the elm tree – *ulmus* in Latin. Meadowsweet, verbena and water-mint were the three herbs held to be most sacred by the Druids, and meadowsweet was used in the Middle Ages as a strewing herb to freshen the stale atmosphere in churches and other public places. Gerard wrote that the scent, 'makes the heart merrie and joyful and delighteth the senses.' The herb was often added to beer or wine and was used to make a type of mead in Chaucer's time. A decoction of the root in wine was considered a specific in the treatment of fevers. During the 19th century, the salicylic component of meadowsweet was the substance originally extracted to create aspirin. The plant's natural balancers mean that it does not have any of the side-effects of the synthesized drug, such as gastric bleeding.

### Parts used

Flowering herb, including leaves.

### Active constituents

Volatile oil, with salicylaldehyde; phenolic glycosides, flavonoids, polyphenolics, tannins, coumarin, ascorbic acid.

### How it works in the body

The salicylic component is responsible for the action of the plant as an anti-inflammatory and painkiller in musculoskeletal disorders, such as arthritis. It is this constituent that is employed in conditions of excess acidity in the digestive system, for example, where there is indigestion caused by the over-production of acid, for stomach ulcers and in irritable bowel syndrome. It is thought not merely to reduce acidity but, where there is inflammation, actively to promote healing in the gut. It has long been used as a gentle remedy for diarrhoea, and was extolled as a specific for children's diarrhoea, a view endorsed by medical herbalists today.

### Applications

Use as an infusion, 200 ml (8 fl oz), three times a day for digestive disorders; use a double-strength infusion and take three times a day for diarrhoea in adults. Take the tincture, 2 ml (40 drops), three times a day for arthritic complaints.

### Indications

• Digestive complaints, especially with acidity, for example, gastric ulcers, irritable bowel syndrome.
• Diarrhoea in adults and children.
• Arthritic complaints.

### Contraindications

Do not take where there is sensitivity to salicylates or allergy to aspirin.

# CLEAVERS
*Rubiaceae* GALIUM APARINE

A common weed, cleavers has long thin stems and rings or whorls of leaves covered in tiny prickles, which catch on clothing, animals, or other plants. The plant grows to about 1.5m (5 ft), and twines itself around and through other plants. The flowers are tiny, white or greenish white, and star-like. It grows throughout Europe and North America, in gardens and hedges and on wasteground.

### History
Many of the common names of this plant describe its clinging nature: cleavers, catchweed, and ever-lasting friendship. The botanical name, *Galium aparine*, is derived from the Greek *galium,* meaning milk, and *aparine* from *aparo,* to seize. The reference to milk alludes to its reputed use as an agent to curdle milk, while 'to seize' refers again to its tenacious character. The stems of the whole plant have reportedly been used in Greece and Sweden as a sieve for milk, and the seeds, dried and slightly roasted, were used as a substitute for coffee in Sweden. Cleavers used to be a favorite ingredient in the old spring tonics made after long winters, when fresh greens were just

reappearing, and it was often used in country areas as a cold remedy. It is said that the roots when eaten by birds tend to tinge their bones red.

### Parts used
Leaves and stems.

### Active constituents
Iridoids, polyphenolic acids, anthra-quinones (roots), alkanes and flavonoids, tannins and coumarins.

### How it works in the body
Cleavers' main action is that of a diuretic. It is prescribed for kidney stones and other urinary com-plaints such as cystitis as a way of eliminating toxins from the body via the urinary system. In addition, its eliminative nature means it is helpful in skin conditions, for example, eczema and psoriasis. It is thought to be an effective lym-phatic cleanser, and is used to treat swollen lymph glands. It is possibly a combination of these detoxifying properties that has promoted its use in cancers and similar illnesses. One of the iridoids acts as a mild laxative. There is some research into its properties with regard to the lowering of blood pressure, and

it has reportedly been helpful as a remedy for insomnia.

### Applications
Cleavers is reportedly at its best for cases of swellings and tumours when taken internally as a juice. To make this, wash the fresh herb and pulp it with water in a food pro-cessor or blender. Strain the juice and drink a wineglassful a day. It is possible to freeze the juice in ice-trays and defrost it as required. It can also be taken as an infusion: 1 cup, 200 ml (8 fl oz), three times a day. Externally, the cooled infusion may be used as a wash or poultice for inflamed skin, and it has been used as a cream or oint-ment for tumours and ulcerations.

### Indications
- Internally, skin conditions such as eczema and psoriasis.
- Externally, for ulceration and tumours.
- Urinary tract complaints, such as kidney stones and cystitis.
- For the nervous system as a sleep-inducing tonic.
- Swollen lymph glands.

### Contraindications
**Do not** use if blood pressure is low.

# GINKGO

*Ginkgoaceae* GINKGO BILOBA (*bai guo*)

Also known as the maidenhair tree, ginkgo is a giant fern, native to China and Japan. It has one or more trunks, and the leaves are notable for their fan-like shape.

### History

Ginkgo is thought to be the oldest living species of tree, with some specimens known to have lived for 1000 years. It was the only growing plant to survive the atomic bomb at Hiroshima. It has been used as a remedy in China for thousands of years, and with current research confirming its use as an agent to improve declining mental faculties, ginkgo is becoming increasingly popular – so much so that it may become an endangered species.

### Parts used

Leaves and seeds.

### Active constituents

Lignans; the ginkgolides (A, B and C), flavonoids, terpenes, essential oil, tannins.

### How it works in the body

The ginkgolides, especially B, work as a platelet activating factor (PAF) antagonist. PAF is involved in initiating both allergic and inflammatory reactions, in particular, asthma. The flavonoid is the agent thought to improve circulation to the brain.

### Applications

Leaves are prepared as an infusion; take 200 ml (8 fl oz), twice a day. Seeds are used as a decoction, 200 ml (8 fl oz); again, take twice a day. Tincture is prepared from the leaves, and for circulatory problems should be taken, 5 ml (1 tsp), three times a day. Tablets are available commercially. Treatment needs to last at least three months to affect improvement in mental faculties. Chinese dosage for the leaves is 3–4.5 g (⅛–¼ oz) and for the seed 4.5–9 g (¼–½ oz).

### Indications

- Circulation, to aid memory, concentration, and in age-related dementia.
- Asthma, particularly in children (use only under the guidance of a medical or herbal practitioner).

### Contraindications

If you are already taking medication for a circulatory-related condition, consult a herbal or medical practitioner before using ginkgo. In asthma cases, **do not** discontinue orthodox medications, and consult a herbal or medical practitioner before using the herb. **Do not** exceed the dose stated, as large amounts can cause adverse reactions. In Chinese medicine ginkgo is considered slightly toxic and only small amounts should be taken for short periods under a qualified practitioner. Symptoms of overdose include headache, tremors, fever and irritability. The antidote is 60 g (3 oz) of *Radix glycyrrhizae uralensis* (*gan cao*) or 30 g (1½ oz) of boiled shells of ginkgo fruit.

### Benefits of ginkgo

*Aids memory and concentration*

*With help from a practitioner in children's asthma*

*Circulatory aid for cold hands and feet*

# LIQUORICE

*Leguminosae* GLYCYRRHIZA GLABRA (*gan cao*)

There are many different species of liquorice, which is a native of southern Europe and Asia. Most have roots that possess a degree of sweetness, but a few are exceptionally sweet and also have medicinal value. The species discussed here grows to about 2 m (6 ft)and has pale yellow flowers.

### History
Liquorice was mentioned by the Greeks in the 3rd century BC, and the botanical name comes from the Greek *glukus*, meaning sweet, and *rhiza*, root. The name, liquorice, derives from the Latin *liquiritia*. The herb was commonly in use in Germany in the Middle Ages, and was cultivated in England in 1562.

### Parts used
Root.

### Active constituents
Triterpenes (mainly glycyrrhizin), flavonoids and isoflavonoids, coumarins, chalcones, polysaccharides, volatile oil, starch and sugars.

### How it works in the body
The glycyrrhizin, which is 50 times sweeter than sugar, is responsible in the main for the plant's function in the respiratory system; it acts as an expectorant and helps to prevent and ease coughing. This ingredient and its derivatives work as anti-inflammatories. It is also largely the glycyrrhizin which gives an anti-allergenic effect, especially when treating asthma. In the digestive system, liquorice is known to have a protective effect on the liver, helping to detoxify and rid the body of unwanted elements. In China it has been used to treat hepatitis and jaundice. The plant is also used to treat nausea, bloating and vomiting, and is a valuable agent in the treatment of stomach ulcers. Liquorice has a beneficial effect on the adrenal glands, supporting them in their function of healing the body. The herb also has immuno-stimulant properties, and possibly anticarcinogenic principles. American research has found that a commercially prepared extract, deglycyrrhizinated liquorice, or DGL, is effective in the treatment of ulcers and less likely to raise blood pressure than the herb itself. Liquorice obtained and prepared at home should still be regarded with caution, since it should not be taken in conditions of high blood pressure.

Chinese properties are sweet and neutral if used raw; sweet and warming if dry-fried before using in a decoction.

### Applications
As a decoction, take 100 ml (4 fl oz) daily for constipation. Take as a tincture, 2 ml (40 drops), twice a day for all other complaints. Make as a syrup to ease sore throats and dry coughs. The Chinese dosage is 2–12 g (⅛–⅜ oz).

### Indications
- Bloating, nausea, indigestion, and also stomach ulcers.
- A gentle laxative.
- Mouthwash for mouth ulcers.
- For dry coughs, and as an expectorant for catarrhal conditions.
- For mild asthma (under the supervision of a qualified medical or herbal practitioner).
- Chest complaints, including bronchitic conditions.
- Arthritis (with inflamed joints).
- To support the adrenal glands.

### Contraindications
**Do not** take liquorice during pregnancy. **Do not** take if suffering from high blood pressure.

# GOLDENSEAL

*Ranunculaceae* HYDRASTIS CANADENSIS

A native of Canada and the eastern United States, this herb is a member of the buttercup family. It grows 15–30 cm (6–12 in) high, with hairy stems leading to two-lobed leaves and small greenish white flowers. It has red fruit and a yellow root.

### History

This plant is known as yellow root or yellow puccoon by Native Americans, but these names were given to other plants as well, so there was initially confusion as to the exact species. It was used as a remedy by the Cherokees and later by settlers, but was not medicinally officially recognized until c.1798.

### Parts used

Rhizome.

### Active constituents

Isoquinoline alkaloids (including hydrastine, berberine and canadine), fatty acids, resin, polyphenolic acids, volatile oil.

### How it works in the body

The isoquinoline alkaloids are thought to be largely responsible for goldenseal's medicinal actions, the hydrastine acting as an astringent and as a hemostatic agent (stops bleeding). The berberine has both antibacterial and amoebicidal properties, while the canadine is thought to stimulate the uterine muscles. Goldenseal's main use is in the treatment of mucous membranes throughout the body. It is used in the respiratory system for conditions of excess mucus and also for the eyes, nose, and throat where inflammation is present. Its antibacterial properties make it useful in combating infection, especially in the mouth or eyes. Used for short periods as a tonic it can increase appetite and stimulate digestion. In the reproductive system it alleviates heavy bleeding and acts as an astringent on the membranes where there is vaginal infection.

### Applications

As a decoction, goldenseal may be used as a gargle or mouthwash, two or three times a day. The powder may be prepared as an infusion for use as a douche in cases of vaginal infections. The tincture may be taken, 1 ml (20 drops), twice daily. A dilute infusion may be used as an eyewash.

### Indications

- Sore throats (gargle); sore gums, mouth ulcers (mouthwash).
- Inflamed or sore eyes (eyewash).
- Stimulate the appetite (tonic).
- Mild laxative (with other herbs).
- Reduces heavy menstrual bleeding.

### Contraindications

**Do not** take in pregnancy or while breastfeeding, since it is a uterine stimulant. **Do not** take in cases of high blood pressure. **Do not** exceed the dosages stated: goldenseal is toxic in large quantities.

### Benefits of goldenseal

Eases symptoms of sinusitis

An eyewash will ease inflammation

Healing for mouth ulcers

Gargle for sore throats

Improves sluggish digestion and aids appetite

# ST JOHN'S WORT

*Hypericaceae* HYPERICUM PERFOLIATUM

This species is native to Europe and Britain and has been imported into North America, where it thrives. Different species grow in many other parts of the world. This hypericum can grow to about 1 m(3 ft) high, and has small green leaves and bright-yellow five-petalled flowers. There are small black dots on the petal margins, underneath which are oil glands.

### History

The name *Hypericum* comes from the Greek *huper*, meaning over, and *eriko*, an apparition, a reference to the herb's reputation for driving out evil spirits. Theplant is known as St John's wort because the first flowers each year are said to open on St John's Day, 24 June. In trials, it has been shown that compared with orthodox antidepressants St John's wort has a similar beneficial effect, with fewer side-effects. Its value as an immune-system herb is being harnessed in conditions such as HIV and other viral illnesses, and research into this aspect continues. Note: Caution is required, since American research has found that some people experienced hyperactivity or numbness in the hands after using the herb.

### Parts used

Whole herb.

### Active constituents

Essential oil, hypericins, flavonoids and epicatechin.

### How it works in the body

St John's wort works primarily in the nervous system, the hypericin in combination with the other constituents acting as an anti-depressant. American studies have found that this herb may be used in combination with *Ginkgo biloba* to increase its antidepressant effectiveness. However, if you wish to combine these herbs, or are already taking prescription antidepressants, it is advisable first to consult your medical or herbal practitioner. St John's wort is also a tonic for the nervous system as a whole, and can be used, for example, in the reproductive system in menopause, where physical changes are aggravated by mental and emotional debility. In the digestive system, the herb is beneficial to the liver, and in the respiratory system the antiviral properties make it especially useful in colds and flus. Its antiviral benefits are helpful in improving the immune system as a whole. Externally, the oil is used as an antiseptic to heal wounds and to ease nerve pain, for example, in shingles and repetitive strain injury.

### Applications

As an infusion, take 200 ml (8 fl oz), twice a day. The tincture should be taken, 2 ml (40 drops), three times a day. Externally, the oil may be applied twice a day (*see* Herbal Methods, nerve tonic oil, p.25). As a cream, apply twice a day to stings or cuts.

### Indications

- Anti-depressant.
- Nervous system tonic.
- Menopause associated with emotional debility.
- Tonic for the digestive system.
- Colds and flu.
- Viral complaints, such as herpes, HIV and AIDS.
- Topically, for shingles and repetitive strain injury.
- For stings or cuts.

### Contraindications

**Do not** exceed the stated dosage. Over-use of this herb can cause photosensitivity in some people.

# LAVENDER

*Labiatae* LAVANDULA OFFICINALIS/ANGUSTIFOLIA

A well-known shrub, lavender is native to western Mediterranean countries but is cultivated worldwide for its fragrance. There are many different species. The grey-green leaves are narrow, and the flowers form a pale to dark purple spike at the end of a tall stalk. It grows to about 1 m (3 ft) in height.

### History

Used by the Romans as a perfume for the bath, the plant possibly derived its name from *lavare*, Latin for 'to wash'. It was introduced into England in about 1568 and taken to America by the Pilgrim Fathers, where it thrived, despite the harsh winters. In Spain and Portugal it was used as a strewing herb for scenting churches on important occasions, and was also burnt to keep evil spirits away. In the Middle Ages it was one of the ingredients of 'four thieves' vinegar', used by grave robbers to ward off the plague. In the 16th century, it was used as a flavouring for food, and lavender conserves were said to comfort the stomach, while the tea was recommended to relieve headache and exhaustion. It is still used in perfumes and cosmetics.

### Parts used

Flowers, essential oil.

### Active constituents

Volatile oil, coumarins, triterpenes.

### How it works in the body

Lavender has a calming and relaxing quality, which makes it suitable for use in the body's many systems. It is helpful in the digestive system, where it is used to calm indigestion and related symptoms such as wind and bloating. In the nervous system, lavender is helpful for headaches, depression and sleeplessness, and it is also used in asthma, where there is a nervous element contributing to the symptoms. Topically, it is added to creams and oils as a rub in arthritic complaints, since it acts as a painkiller, relieving painful joints. For neuralgia or nerve pain, it is used externally in creams and oils.

### Applications

For indigestion, as an infusion, take 100 ml (4 fl oz), twice daily. For sleeplessness, as a tincture, take 2½–5 ml (½–1 tsp), at night. Add lavender infusion or essential oil to a bath before bedtime to relieve stress and tension, or use in a diffuser to aid sleep. For headaches, add two drops of lavender essential oil to a bowl of cold water and soak a cloth to make a compress to place across the forehead. Five drops of lavender oil added to a footbath relieves exhaustion. As a rub for arthritic complaints, add one drop each of lavender essential oil and wintergreen essential oil to 50 ml (4 tbsp) of a carrier oil. The essential oil can be used neat on insect bites or stings.

### Indications

- Indigestion, wind, and bloating.
- Insomnia.
- Nervous complaints, including stress, tension, headaches.
- Arthritic complaints.
- Neuralgia.
- Insect bites and stings.

### Contraindications

**Never** take essential oils internally. **Do not** add them to a baby's bath, since he or she might ingest the oils by sucking their fingers.

# MOTHERWORT

*Labiatae* LEONURUS CARDIACA (*yi mu cao*)

Chinese pharmaceutical name: *herba leonuri heterophylli*

A native of Europe, this herb is naturalized in other countries, including England and North America. It reaches a height of about 1m (3ft) and has dull green hairy leaves and clusters of pink flowers. Although found mainly on wasteground, it is sometimes cultivated in gardens. Another variety, *Leonurus hetrophyllus*, is used in Chinese herbalism in the same way as *cardiaca*.

### History

The botanical name comes from the Greek words for lion's tail and *cardiaca*, which refers to the heart. This name indicates its traditional use as a herbal remedy for palpitations, especially of a nervous origin. In old herbals it was often referred to as a tonic both to strengthen the heart and to relieve stress placed on the heart by nervous disorders. Culpeper wrote, '. . . there is no better herb to drive melancholy vapours from the heart.'

### Parts used

Whole herb.

### Active constituents

Iridoids, diterpenes, flavonoids and caffeic acid.

### How it works in the body

As its history indicates, motherwort is a remedy for the cardiovascular system, particularly where there are palpitations aggravated by nervous tension or stress. Its actions are antispasmodic and sedative, helping to regulate the heart, and also acting as a tonic to strengthen weakness of the heart. It can be used where there is high blood pressure. In addition, in the reproductive system, it helps to bring on a delayed period by stimulating the uterine muscles. It is also used where there is premenstrual syndrome, especially in early menopause. In Chinese herbalism, its use in the reproductive system extends from irregular periods and premenstrual pain, to a treatment for infertility and immobile abdominal masses. The Chinese properties are acrid, bitter and slightly cold.

### Applications

Take an infusion, 200 ml (8 fl oz), twice daily. For the tincture, take 2 ml (40 drops) three times a day. The Chinese dosage is 9–60 g (½–3 oz).

### Indications

- Palpitations associated with nervous tension and stress.
- Tonic for the heart.
- High blood pressure.
- PMS, especially in menopause.

### Contraindications

**Do not** take motherwort during pregnancy. This is confirmed in Chinese cautions. **Do not** take in reproductive conditions where there is a tendency to heavy periods.

# HONEYSUCKLE

*Caprifoliaceae* LONICERA SPECIES *(jin yin hua)*

Chinese pharmaceutical name: *flos lonicerae japonicae*

Honeysuckle is a European native, but it is grown extensively throughout the world, especially in China, and there are many species. In Europe, the most common is *Lonicera caprifolium*, while in China it is *Lonicera japonica*. It is a climbing shrub, growing to some 4 m (13 ft). It has oval leaves, which grow opposite each other, and yellow flowers either tinged with orange (*caprifolium*) or white (*japonica*). The flowers give way to red berries.

### History

Culpeper said, 'The leaves, which are the only part used, are sometimes put into gargarisms for sore throats . . . Some command a decoction of them for a cough.' The herbalist Gerard wrote in the 16th century, 'The floures steeped in oile and set in the Sun, are good to annoint the body that is benummed, and growne very cold.' The family name *Lonicera* was given by Carl Linnaeus, the Swedish botanist who originated the system of botanical naming, in honor of Adam Lonicer, who wrote many botanical books. *Lonicera japonica* was first mentioned in the *Tang Materia Medica*.

### Parts used
Flowers and leaves.

### Active constituents
Volatile oil, luteolin, inositol and tannins.

### How it works in the body
Western applications of *Lonicera caprifolium* tend to follow the age-old usage: that is, the leaves are used as a gargle or mouthwash for sore throats and gum problems, while the flowers are commonly used in treatments for asthma, where they relax the airways. The Chinese usage of *Lonicera japonica* is much more extensive, and research has shown an antibacterial action against both *streptococcus* and *staphylococcus* bacteria. In laboratory experiments, some protective effects on the lungs have been demonstrated in cases of tuberculosis. Traditional Chinese applications include cases of abscesses or swellings, especially of the breast, throat, eyes or internally. It is employed in the early stages of diseases accompanied by fever, sensitivity to wind, sore throat and headache and is also used in cases of damp-heat dysenteric disorders, or painful urinary dysfunction. The Chinese properties are sweet and cold.

### Applications
Use internally as an infusion, 200 ml (8 fl oz), twice daily. Use the infusion as a gargle or mouthwash, twice daily (*see* Herbal Methods, gargles and mouthwashes, p.21). Chinese dosage is 9–15 g (½–¾ oz).

### Indications
- Sore throats and gum problems.
- Asthma (under the supervision of a qualified herbal or medicinal practitioner).
- Infections accompanied by fever, sore throat, headache.
- Abscesses or swellings, especially of the breast or throat.
- Dysentery or painful urinary dysfunction.

### Contraindications
The berries should not be taken, since they are poisonous. The Chinese cautions indicate that this remedy should not be used in cases of diarrhoea. It is also contraindicated for sores where there is *qi* (energy) deficiency, as demonstrated by a clear discharge.

# LYCIUM FRUIT

*Solanaceae* LYCIUM CHINENSE *(gou qi zi)*

Chinese pharmaceutical name: *fructus lycii*

This shrub is native to, and widely cultivated throughout, China. It grows to about 4 m (12 ft) and bears distinctive, bright red berries.

### History

The plant was first mentioned medicinally in AD 1 in the *Divine Husbandman's Classic of the Materia Medica* and is also known as Chinese wolfberry fruit and matrimony vine fruit. It has been used medicinally for thousands of years. Research has shown that the herb has a protective effect on the liver, and also aids its recovery from the effects of toxicity. In laboratory conditions it was demonstrated to be effective in breaking down lipids. It has further been shown to lower blood pressure and ease breathing. In folk medicine it has been used for disorders where wasting and thirst are features.

### Parts used

Berries and root.

### Active constituents

Betaine, carotene, physalien, thiamine, riboflavin, vitamin C, beta-sitosterol and linoleic acid.

### How it works in the body

The berries are thought to have a protective effect on the liver and kidneys, nourishing and acting as a tonic. Conditions where this is most effective are those where there is a sore back and legs; low-grade abdominal pain; excessive urination at night (nocturia); wasting and thirsting disorders; consumption; and, in the reproductive system for men, impotence. Another of its major functions is as a tonic for the eyes, especially where the circulation is thought to be poor, in conditions of dizziness, blurred vision and diminished sight. In the respiratory system it is used to tone up the lungs, especially where there is a consumptive cough. In the cardiovascular system, as a circulatory tonic, it helps to reduce blood pressure and to lower lipid levels. The Chinese properties are those of sweet and neutral.

### Applications

Both berries and root are made as a decoction, 200 ml (8 fl oz), a day. A tincture of the root can be made, take 5 ml (1 tsp), twice daily. The Chinese dosage is 6–18 g (⅕–⅞ oz).

### Indications

- Tonic for the liver and kidney.
- Improves circulation, reduces high blood pressure, and lowers lipid levels.
- Where wasting and thirst are a feature, such as in diabetes.
- Consumptive coughs.
- Tonic for the eyes.
- Tonic for male impotence.

### Contraindications

Chinese cautions indicate that this herb should not be used in cases of digestive weakness where the stools are loose.

---

### Benefits of lycium fruit

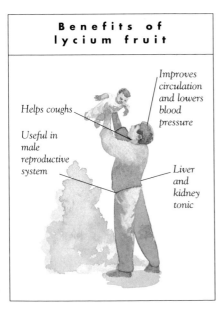

Improves circulation and lowers blood pressure

Helps coughs

Useful in male reproductive system

Liver and kidney tonic

# LEMON BALM

*Labiatae* MELISSA OFFICINALIS

Common in Europe, Britain, Asia, North Africa, and North America, lemon balm can grow to about 1.2 m (4 ft) high. The oval leaves have serrated edges and occur in pairs along the stem; when crushed, they emit a lemony aroma. The white flowers are borne in the axils of the leaves.

### History

Lemon balm is a bee plant, the Greek name *Melissa* actually meaning bee. Balm comes from the word balsam, meaning balm for your sorrows. Gerard said 'It is profitably planted where bees are kept', while John Evelyn wrote, 'Balm is sovereign for the brain, strengthening the memory and powerfully chasing away melancholy.' Lemon balm combined with nutmeg, angelica and lemon peel was known as Carmelite water, and was used as a remedy for nervous headaches and neuralgia.

### Parts used

Leaves and flowers, essential oil.

### Active constituents

Volatile oil, flavonoids, polyphenolics (including rosmarinic acid) and triterpenic acids.

### How it works in the body

In the nervous system, the oil is the main agent used to calm and soothe and has a relaxant effect on the muscles. This has been supported by research, where *Melissa* has been used in states of excitability, palpitations, depression, and headache. The polyphenolics, especially the rosmarinic acid, are responsible for an antiviral action. A cream made from lemon balm has been shown to be effective against herpes simplex, more commonly known as cold sores; the duration of the outbreaks has been halved and the outbreaks themselves become less frequent. Lemon balm also has an action on the thyroid, reducing over-activity of the gland (hyperthyroidism). In the reproductive system, this herb has been used in the menopause to ease symptoms, including hot flushes and anxiety, and to regulate periods, as well as to alleviate period pains.

### Applications

Use as an infusion, 200 ml (8 fl oz), three times a day in states of nervous excitability and headaches. Use the tincture, 3 ml (60 drops), twice a day internally for viral complaints. Prepare as a cream or ointment to use topically on cold sores (*see* Herbal Methods pp.26–27). Use the essential oil in an oil burner to uplift the spirits, or add to a bath to relieve stress and tension.

### Indications

- Nervous complaints.
- Internally (tincture) for viral complaints, such as cold sores, shingles, colds and flu.
- Externally for cold sores.
- In menopause, to ease symptoms.
- To help regulate periods and alleviate period pain.

### Contraindications

**Do not** use the oil internally. **Do not** add the oil to a baby's bath, since he or she can ingest it by sucking their fingers.

# PEPPERMINT

*Labiatae* MENTHA PIPERITA *(bo he)*

Chinese pharmaceutical name: *herba menthae haplocalycis*

A native of Europe, mint is perhaps one of the best-known culinary herbs. The medicinal variety is a hybrid – a naturally occurring cross of watermint and spearmint. There are two types, black and white peppermint, which are widely cultivated, in particular in North America. The plant grows to about 40 cm (16 in) in height and the green leaves, with a serrated edge, give off the familiar mint odour when crushed between the fingers; it bears small, reddish-purple flowers.

### History

According to Vogel, wild mint was used by Native American tribes in the Missouri Valley as a carminative, and by many other tribes to alleviate fevers.

### Parts used

Leaves, essential oil.

### Active constituents

Essential oil, up to 1.5 per cent, containing menthol, flavonoids and rosmarinic acid.

### How it works in the body

The menthol in the oil is responsible for an antiseptic effect on the body as a whole. The leaves, with their combination of constituents, are useful in the treatment of digestive disorders, having an antispasmodic effect which is calming on the gut, especially where there is gastric upset due to over-indulgence. It is also used in complaints such as irritable bowel syndrome, gastritis and where there is excess wind and colic. It has a diaphoretic element which encourages sweating, so has been used in colds and flu to bring down a fever. In Chinese medicine it is also used to disperse fever, headaches and coughs, and is used in the early stages of colds and flu. Additionally, the Chinese use it for rashes, for example in measles, since it encourages the rash to progress, thereby speeding recovery. It can also act as a painkiller when applied externally. The oil has antibacterial properties. The Chinese properties are acrid, aromatic and cooling.

### Applications

As an infusion, 200 ml (8 fl oz) of peppermint can be taken three times a day after meals to aid the digestion.

In colds and flu, add a pinch of the herb to a tea made of equal parts of yarrow and elderflower to relieve symptoms. Take as a tincture, 1 ml (20 drops), three times a day for digestive problems. Add to the decoction five minutes before finishing; it must not be overcooked. Externally, mix 10 drops of the oil in 50 ml (4 tbsp) of carrier oil and rub it on inflamed joints. Peppermint capsules are available on prescription only. The Chinese dosage is 1.5–6 g (¹⁄₁₆– ¼ oz).

### Indications

- Irritable bowel syndrome, gastritis, excess wind, and colic.
- Colds and flu – add a pinch to other herbal remedies to help reduce a fever.
- Externally, use the oil to relieve the plain of inflamed joints.

### Contraindications

**Do not** use peppermint for children under the age of 12, either as an infusion or topically as an essential oil. **Do not** take the essential oil internally. The Chinese cautions recommend that this herb should not be given to nursing mothers as it may stem milkflow. Also, take care in weakness or prolonged fevers.

# PASSION FLOWER

*Passifloraceae* PASSIFLORA INCARNATA

Passion flower is native to the southern United States and also to Central and South America; it is also cultivated in many other countries. The plant is a climber, with curling tendrils, which can reach up to 9 m (30 ft) in length. The striking flowers give way to large oval, orange berries. There are many different species of the plant, which flourishes in sunny locations where there is rich soil.

### History

The name passion flower refers to the Passion, or Crucifixion, of Christ in the Christian tradition. The flower's central corona is thought to resemble Christ's crown of thorns, while the five stamens are linked to the five wounds, and the three styles to the nails. It was listed in the herbals of the Aztecs as an emetic and purgative, and the Mayas used it for swellings and for ringworm. Native Americans traditionally used it for its sedative qualities for restlessness, insomnia, and in the treatment of neuralgia; it has also been used for epilepsy.

### Parts used

Leaves.

### Active constituents

Alkaloids (some of which have not been fully verified), flavonoids (including apigenin, an 8-pyrone derivative), sterols and sugars.

### How it works in the body

Passiflora is primarily a sedative, acting on the central nervous system through the combined actions of the alkaloids, flavonoids, and the 8-pyrone derivative, but the mechanisms by which this works have not yet been extensively researched. Its sedative qualities have been used in overactive states ranging from epilepsy to neuralgia and anxiety. It is extremely helpful in combating sleeplessness. One flavonoid, apigenin, is known to have antispasmodic and anti-inflammatory action, which has been used in the cardiovascular system to ease high blood pressure and to quiet palpitations. In other systems it is used to ease muscle spasm.

### Applications

As an infusion, take 200–400 ml (8–16 fl oz) daily. As a tincture, take 2 ml (40 drops) three times a day, or 5 ml (1 tsp) at night for insomnia. The herb is also available commercially as tablets.

### Indications

- Insomnia.
- Anxiety, states of restlessness, panic attacks.
- Neuralgia, as a mild painkiller.
- High blood pressure.
- Relaxant in diverticulitis and irritable bowel syndrome.
- To relax the airways.
- Period and ovarian pain.

### Contraindications

**Do not** use during pregnancy. Large doses can lead to a soporific state.

### Benefits of passion flower

- Useful in insomnia
- Relieves anxiety and panic attacks
- Relaxes digestion in irritable bowel syndrome
- Mild painkiller for neuralgia

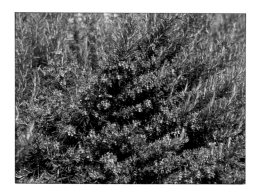

# ROSEMARY
*Labiatae* ROSMARINUS OFFICINALIS

This plant is well known as a culinary herb, and although a native of Mediterranean regions it is widely cultivated in gardens in many parts of the world. As a shrub, it grows to about 2 m (6 ft) high and has woody stems, narrow, needlelike leaves and pale lilac or blue flowers. The scent is distinctive.

### History
The use of rosemary for improving the memory has a long history. For this reason, it was often included in a wedding bouquet as a floral emblem of love and fidelity. Sir Thomas More wrote, 'I lett it runne all over my garden walls, not onlie because my bees love it, but because it is the herb sacred to remembrance and, therefore, to friendship.' It was also traditionally grown in gardens where the woman ruled the household. In earlier time, rosemary was burnt as an incense to cleanse the air in sickrooms and, together with rue, it was placed in courtrooms to offset contagion from prisoners who had been held in jails. The name *Rosmarinus* comes from the Latin meaning dew of the sea, a reference to its refreshing effect on the spirit.

### Parts used
Leaves, essential oil.

### Active constituents
Volatile oil, flavonoids, including apigenin and diosmetin, rosmarinic acid and other phenolic acids, diterpenes, triterpenes, including ursolic acid.

### How it works in the body
One of rosemary's primary actions is that of an anti-inflammatory and tonic, which is thought to be due to combined constituents, including the apigenin, rosmarinic, and ursolic acids. The diosmetin is known to help in strengthening the capillaries, which is makes it valuable in the cardiovascular system, where rosemary is used to improve circulation and raise low blood pressure. This circulatory effect is particularly directed at the circulation to the head, which is thought to contribute to improving the memory and concentration. It is also used in cases of Raynaud's Syndrome, a condition of poor circulation in the hands and feet. Rosemary is helpful where there is listlessness and depression, and so can improve states of lethargy and debility.

### Applications
The infusion can be taken internally, 200 ml (8 fl oz), daily. Externally, use the infusion as a rinse for the hair to improve circulation to the scalp. It can also be added to the bath as a refreshing way to start the day. The tincture can be taken, 2 ml (40 drops), twice a day. Add the essential oil to bathwater or use it in a diffuser; it is helpful for concentration and to aid studying.

### Indications
- Improves circulation to the brain to aid memory and concentration.
- Cold hands and feet.
- Low blood pressure.
- States of debility.
- As a hair rinse to improve the scalp and encourage hair growth.

### Contraindications
This herb should **not** be used where there is high blood pressure.

# YELLOW DOCK

*Polygonaceae* RUMEX CRISPUS

The large leaves of this dock are similar to those of other docks, except that the edges are extremely furled, giving rise to its other common name, curled dock. It is mainly found in wasteland and by the side of roads. It originated in Europe and Africa, but has now been transplanted to many other parts of the world.

### History

Along with others in the same family, this herb is known for its cleansing properties and has long been used to help rid the system of toxins; Culpeper recommended it for expelling damaging 'cholers' from the body. He went on to say, 'the yellow dock root is best to be taken when either the blood or the liver is affected by choler.' This may explain its use in the past for treatment of various types of cancer. The leaves used to be eaten as part of a spring tonic, but research has shown them to have large quantities of oxalates, which are implicated in causing kidney stones and gout. The root, however, does not cause this problem in the dosages given. According to Vogel, the European species of dock was one of the few herbs adopted into Native American usage, alongside the indigenous varieties. The Dakotas used the leaves as a poultice to relieve boils, while the roots were used for their tannins by the Ojibwas for closing and healing cuts. In Chinese medicine it is used for constipation, boils and fungal infections.

### Parts used

Root.

### Active constituents

Anthraquinone glycosides, tannins, rumicin and oxalates.

### How it works in the body

The anthraquinones are responsible for the laxative effect for which this herb is mainly employed. They work by stimulating the colon to expel waste and toxins. In small amounts, anything which has a laxative effect may be cleansing for the body, but large amounts would have a purgative effect, causing excessive peristalsis, resulting in griping pains. However, at the right dosage the plant gives a gentle action well suited to relieving moderate constipation. It also acts to aid the digestive processes. Combined with other herbs, yellow dock is well suited to assist the liver in the cleansing of toxins from the skin, and it is used in complaints such as eczema, psoriasis and acne. In the musculoskeletal system, where there is often a build-up of toxins resulting from constipation, the herb is again cleansing.

### Applications

The root is usually made into a decoction. Take 100 ml (4 fl oz) daily for short periods for constipation. For skin problems, combine it with marigold and cleavers and use 100 ml (4 fl oz) daily. As a tincture, take 2½ ml (50 drops) three times a day.

### Indications

- Clears constipation and aids the digestion.
- Skin complaints, such as eczema, psoriasis and acne.
- Arthritic complaints.
- To clear fungal infections.

### Contraindications

**Do not** take during pregnancy or while breastfeeding.

*133*

# SAGE

*Labiatae* SALVIA OFFICINALIS

Garden, or red sage as it is also called, comes from countries bordering the Mediterranean and is widely cultivated in many other countries throughout the world. There are many species, but red sage is the medicinal herb. It grows to about 60 cm (2 ft) high, with paired, wrinkled, reddish purple leaves; the flowers are also reddish purple. When crushed, the leaves have a distinctive odour.

### History

*Salvia* comes from the Latin *salvus*, safe, a reference to the plant's long history of medicinal use. In the Middle Ages a popular adage was *Cur mariatur homo cui salvia crescit in horto?*, which translates as 'Why should a man die while sage grows in his garden?' Various superstitions surround the herb; for instance, it is said that where sage grows, prosperity in business matters follows. In France, sage is believed to ease grief and it is often sown in graveyards. Some species have been used as a substitute for tea, and on some Greek islands the leaves are made into sweets. It has also been taken as snuff, and powdered to make a paste similar to toothpaste for whitening the teeth. According

to Vogel, the Lower California Indians ground the seeds of sage and stirred in water to prevent dryness of the mouth and throat. The roots were used by the Catawbas in an ointment for sores.

### Parts used

Leaves.

### Active constituents

Volatile oil with thujone, cineole, borneol and camphor, diterpene bitters, flavonoids, phenolic acids (for example, rosmarinic acid) and salviatannin.

### How it works in the body

It is the thujone that is mainly responsible for sage's antiseptic properties, which make it invaluable as a gargle and mouthwash. It also acts as a circulatory and mild digestive stimulant. In the reproductive system, sage can be used to bring on a delayed period, and in menopause can be taken to relieve sweats and to balance hormonal changes. Sage has also been incorporated in herbal cigarettes to alleviate asthma, the rosmarinic acid acting as an anti-inflammatory and antispasmodic.

### Applications

Take sage as an infusion, 200 ml (8 fl oz), a day, or use as a gargle or mouthwash, 100 ml (4 fl oz), two or three times a day. (*See* Herbal Methods, gargles and mouthwashes p.21). The tincture can be taken, 2 ml (40 drops), twice a day.

### Indications

- As a mouthwash, for sore or bleeding gums and for mouth ulcers. As a gargle, for sore throats, tonsillitis, and similar problems. Also use as a breath freshener.
- To aid circulation and stimulate digestion.
- To bring on a delayed period.
- In menopause, to relieve sweats and balance hormones.

### Contraindications

**Do not** take during pregnancy.

# ELDERFLOWER

*Caprifoliaceae* SAMBUCUS NIGRA

The elder tree is common in Europe and Britain, growing in woods and on wasteground, and it is now also widely found in other parts of the world. When flowering, the tree is a mass of creamy white, flat-topped blossoms, which are followed by large bunches of black berrylike fruits.

### History

The name *Sambucus* comes from the Greek *sambuke*, a musical instrument which is made from the wood of the tree; *nigra* refers to the black berries. The elder tree has possibly more folklore associated with it than any other plant – nearly every country has legends that include it. The ancient Greeks and many other peoples assigned magic powers to it. The English diarist John Evelyn recommended an infusion of elderflowers in vinegar to be added to salads for medicinal benefit. The berries were also made into wine as a tonic for colds and flu, to be taken at bedtime. The Native American Iroquois, and also the Menominees, used an infusion of either the berries or the inner bark of *Sambucus canadensis* as a treatment for fever, to induce sweating, and also as a painkiller. The Meskwakis used it to loosen phlegm in the respiratory tract.

### Parts used

Flowers, berries, leaves, bark.

### Active constituents

Triterpenes (including ursolic acid), fixed oils, flavonoids, phenolic acids.

### How it works in the body

Generally, elderflower has a anti-inflammatory action, attributed to the presence of the ursolic acid. The benefits are mainly directed at the respiratory system; it is a specific for nasal catarrh. It is also useful for allergies such as hayfever and allergic rhinitis. The herb has a diaphoretic effect, encouraging the loss of toxins through sweating, so is particularly useful in colds and flu, where it will lower a fever and reduce excess catarrh. It will, in addition, relieve earache due to the build-up of mucus, and is also good as a gargle for sore throats. Finally, the plant works on the urinary system, having a mild diuretic effect, encouraging the elimination of waste material, which is helpful in arthritic conditions.

### Applications

Use the flowers as an infusion for colds and flu, drinking 200 ml (8 fl oz) three times a day. Use the flowers also as a tincture in allergic as well as arthritic conditions, taking 5 ml (1 tsp) three times a day. The berries can be prepared by decoction. Being rich in vitamin C, they are beneficial for colds and flu – take 200 ml (8 fl oz) twice a day. The leaves are made into an infusion, which can be used as a gargle or mouthwash, and the bark is made into a decoction for the same purpose. (Take only small amounts of bark from the tree or it may be damaged beyond recovery.) Elder leaves have been used as an ointment for chilblains, wounds and dry skin. An infusion of the flowers in the bath will soothe dry skin and act as an inhalant to clear blocked sinuses.

### Indications

- Coughs and colds, to promote the dispersal of catarrh.
- Gargle for sore throats.
- Soothe dry skin.
- Healing agent for chilblains and wounds.
- Arthritic conditions.

# SKULLCAP

*Labiatae* SCUTELLARIA LATERIFLORA

Native to North America, skullcap is also found in Europe, but the species is not thought to have the same medicinal qualities as its New World counterpart. The plant grows to about 60 cm (2 ft) and has thin, square stems with paired leaves covered with fine hairs growing around the stem. The blue flowers are followed by seed capsules shaped like a cap, and it is they that give the herb its name. Skullcap thrives in damp surroundings and is generally found alongside rivers and streams.

### History

One of this plant's common names, mad dog skullcap, refers to its traditional use in North America as a treatment for rabies. It is also known as Virginian skullcap, after the state where it grows abundantly. Among Native Americans, this herb was predominantly used for the reproductive system, to relieve symptoms of premenstrual syndrome. In the 19th century, skullcap's properties and effects on the nervous system were extolled, and the plant became a cure-all for disorders connected with this system, including hysteria, chorea (St Vitus's Dance) and epilepsy. Today's usage confirms its role in the treatment of ailments of the nervous system, although skullcap is perhaps not quite the cure-all it was once thought to be.

### Parts used

Whole herb.

### Active constituents

Flavonoid glycoside, scutellarin, iridoids, volatile oils and waxes, tannins.

### How it works in the body

Skullcap acts as a sedative, both mentally and physically, to calm and sustain an over-excited nervous system, and can be used in cases of stress and tension. Some species have been found to have constituents with anti-inflammatory and antiallergenic properties, and it is possible this extends to *Scutelleria lateriflora*, but further research has yet to be carried out. One species found in China appears to have a beneficial effect in liver disorders such as hepatitis, actually improving liver function. Skullcap's sedative effect helps to alleviate period or ovarian pain.

### Applications

Skullcap may be taken as an infusion, 200 ml (8 fl oz), three times a day. The tincture is taken, 2 ml (40 drops), three times a day.

### Indications

- In conditions of stress and anxiety.
- Included with other herbs such as lavender and passion flower in a remedy for insomnia.
- Ovarian and period pain.

---

### Benefits of skullcap

Restorative in stress and anxiety

Use with passion flower for insomnia

Mild painkiller for period pains

# SAW PALMETTO

*Palmaceae* SERENOA SERRULATA SABAL SERRULATA

This plant originates in North America, more particularly in the Atlantic coastal region, including South Carolina and Florida, and southern California. It is a palm with large prickly, fan-shaped leaves that grows to about 3 m (9 ft). The flowers are pale and the fruit a deep reddish brown.

### History

The Native Americans have a long history of usage of this and related species of palm for medicinal purposes, and the Mayas used *Sabal japa* extensively. The inner bark was made into a decoction and then employed to treat dysentery, abdominal pains and snake and insect bites. In addition, a poultice of the bark was used topically for ulcers. The Houma Indians apparently drank the decoction for kidney problems, while the dried root was used to treat high blood pressure. Vogel lists sources which tell of early settlers using the palm branches to make brooms. Some early settlers apparently saw animals thriving on a diet of the berries and added them to their medicinal stores. Further research is needed into the extensive properties of this plant.

### Parts used
Berries.

### Active constituents
Essential oil, fixed oil, sterols and polysaccharides.

### How it works in the body
As the early settlers discovered, saw palmetto is a tonic which builds and restores body tissue. The sterols have an anabolic action, which helps to build-up and maintain weight, so can usefully be given to those who are convalescing or have lost weight through illness or debility. In the reproductive system it has useful applications for both men and women. In men, it is given to enhance the sex drive and to treat impotence and infertility. In women, it is thought to have an estrogenic action and can be taken where this is a cause of disorder in the reproductive system. As a urinary tract tonic it is used where there is weakness in the neck of the bladder, and also as a diuretic to improve urinary flow. Saw palmetto has been shown to be effective in treating enlargement of the prostate in men.

### Applications
The infusion may be taken, 100 ml (4 fl oz), twice daily. The tincture may be taken, 2 ml (40 drops), three times a day.

### Indications
- In convalescence or debility to restore weight and improve vitality.
- For men, to enhance the sex drive and to treat impotence and infertility.
- For women, to restore estrogenic levels.
- As a diuretic to improve urinary flow.
- For enlargement of the prostate.

# CHICKWEED
*Caryophyllaceae* STELLARIA MEDIA

Acommon garden weed which originated in Europe, chickweed now grows extensively all over the world. The plant, which grows close to the ground, has dark green, oval leaves and tiny white starlike flowers, which give it its botanical name.

### History
As a food the leaves have been used fresh in salads, and as a source of vitamin C – at one time it was recommended for use against scurvy. When boiled as a vegetable, it resembles spinach in taste and texture, and it was often added to soups. Chickweed had a reputation for aiding weight loss, possibly due to its property as a lymph cleanser. In addition, at one time it was used as a treatment for rabies. The plant has been highly valued by herbalists from the time of Gerard and Culpeper to the present.

### Parts used
The leaves and flowers together.

### Active constituents
Saponin glycosides, coumarins, flavonoids, carboxylic acids, triterpenoids and vitamin C.

### How it works in the body
Chickweed is particularly noted for its cooling qualities, and is especially soothing when applied to skin problems presenting as hot and itchy. It is thought the saponins are responsible for relief of the itching. Applied to wounds, it is believed to reduce scarring. In addition, the combined constituents are thought to be beneficial for arthritic conditions, while topically the whole plant has a soothing, healing effect. In small amounts, the herb works also on the digestive system, helping to soothe and heal complaints of the digestive tract.

### Applications
Internally, as an infusion, take 200 ml (8 fl oz) twice a day. Externally, the infusion can be used in the bath to reduce inflammation. Use as a cream or ointment twice a day for skin complaints, or as a poultice if required. It is thought that the fresh herb is better for creams, ointments and poultices than the dried variety. The cream is best kept in the refrigerator, which will enhance its cooling qualities. As a tincture, use internally, 1 ml (20 drops), three times a day.

### Indications
- Internally for eczema, psoriasis and related irritative skin complaints.
- Externally as a cream or ointment to reduce scarring on new wounds.
- As a poultice for boils and abscesses.
- Internally for arthritis complaints, where there is pain and stiffness.
- As a tea for sore throats and coughs, generally healing and cleansing to the lungs.
- For the digestive system gently to encourage calming and healing of the gut.

### Contraindications
This herb may have a laxative effect in large doses. **Avoid** during pregnancy.

# COMFREY

*Boraginaceae* SYMPHYTUM OFFICINALE

The main feature of this plant is the leaves, which are large, oval and bristly. The plant is particularly common on marshy or damp ground and grows to about 1 m (3 ft) high. It bears drooping bell-like flowers, which are either white or purple. The herb originated in Europe and parts of Asia, but today it is also found in North America and Australia.

### History

The name comfrey comes from *con firma*, meaning to join bones, while the botanical name *Symphytum* comes from the Greek meaning to unite bones.

### Parts used

Leaf, internally. Root, externally.

### Active constituents

Allantoin, pyrrolizidine alkaloids, phenolic acids including rosmarinic, mucilage, volatile oil, tannins, and saponins.

### How it works in the body

The principal ingredient allantoin works to promote the healing of tissues within the body. It is complemented by the rosmarinic acid, an anti-inflammatory agent. The mucilage is demulcent and helps to soothe irritative conditions both internally and externally. The tannins act as an astringent. The pyrrolizidine alkaloids, which are concentrated mainly in the root of the plant, are thought to be damaging to the liver. There is, therefore, common agreement by the main bodies of herbal practitioners that the root should not be taken internally. It has, however, been substantiated that the leaf does not present this problem and it may be taken internally under the guidance of a qualified herbal or medical practitioner. Both leaf and root can safely be used externally.

### Applications

The leaf may be made as a tincture, and used under the direction of a herbal or medical practitioner for the purpose of healing stomach ulcers and other disorders, and in the respiratory system for conditions such as bronchitis. The leaf may also be made as a poultice or compress and applied to sprains or bruised areas. It is also possible to make an infused oil from the leaf, which may be applied to the skin over an area where fractures or a break in the bone has occurred, and to scar tissue. Comfrey-infused oil can be used as a massage oil to relieve stiff and aching joints in arthritic conditions. In all these instances, comfrey ointment may be used instead of the oil .

### Indications

- The tincture, under supervision, for stomach ulcers and irritable bowel syndrome and also for bronchitic conditions.
- The oil or ointment for all cases of injury, sprains, breaks and bruises.
- The oil may be rubbed into the skin over arthritic joints.
- The oil on scar tissue, to aid healing.

### Contraindications

**Never** take the leaf internally without the supervision of a qualified herbal or medical practitioner. **Never** apply any comfrey preparations to an open wound, cut or graze. **Never** take the root internally.

# FEVERFEW

*Compositae* TANACETUM PARTHENIUM

This herb grows to about 60 cm (2 ft). The flowers are daisy-like in appearance, with yellow central florets surrounded by an outer ring of white ray florets. They differ from those on other camomiles in that the central disk is almost flat, rather than conical. The leaves are alternate, yellowish green and fernlike. The plant is native to southern Europe, but has spread widely to many parts of the world, including North America.

### History

Feverfew is a corruption of the word febrifuge – an agent used to bring down fever. *Parthenium* derives from the Greek *pyrethrum*, meaning fire, which some say refers to the hotness of the root, while others maintain that it alludes to the heat or burning associated with a fever. Traditionally, the herb was planted in gardens surrounding dwellings to purify the air and ward off disease. This may be due in part to its reputation as an insect repellent. The tincture was used as a wash to alleviate the pain of insect bites and stings, and, if applied to exposed skin, the diluted tincture was said to be effective in keeping off insects.

### Parts used

Leaves.

### Active constituents

Volatile oil containing spiroketal enol ethers; sesquiterpene lactones including parthenolide; acetylene derivatives, mainly in the root.

### How it works in the body

Feverfew's action against fevers is thought to be due to the sesquiterpene lactones, which inhibit the release of arachidonic acid in the body. These ingredients have also been shown to inhibit other substances that contribute to preventing blood from clotting. In the reproductive system, feverfew has long had the function of promoting menstrual flow. Its main use today is to prevent and alleviate headaches, especially migraine. Research indicates that the sesquiterpene lactones, among other constituents, inhibit the secretion of serotonin, which is implicated in the onset of migraine. Another area of research is studying the role of feverfew in the musculoskeletal system, where its inhibitory effects are thought to help control pain in conditions such as arthritis.

### Applications

The fresh leaf is taken as a preventative. Two leaves daily may be taken, wrapped in a piece of bread. The tincture may be taken, ½ ml (10 drops), once a day. Tablets and capsules are available commercially.

### Indications

- To reduce fevers.
- To promote menstrual flow.
- To prevent and also to alleviate headaches, especially migraine.
- A painkiller, with other herbs, in arthritic conditions.

### Contraindications

**Do not** take in pregnancy. **Do not** take this herb if you are receiving medication such as Warfarin which thins the blood. The fresh leaf should only be taken with bread or similar substances, since it may cause ulcers if it comes into contact with the mucous membranes in the mouth.

# PAO D'ARCO

*Bignoniaceae* TABEBUIA SPECIES

There are many different species of Pao d'Arco (the plant's Portuguese name), or lapacho (its Spanish name). It is a tree which originates in Brazil but has now spread to other countries in South America and to North America. The tree grows to about 30 m (100 ft), and has pinkish purple flowers.

### History

One of the many species of Pao d'Arco, also commonly known as taheebo, is frequently grown as an ornamental garden tree in North America. The species are difficult to distinguish and there is some dispute as to which have the specified medicinal qualities. *Tabebuia avellanedae* and *Tabebuia impetignosa* are most commonly used medicinally. Pao d'Arco has been used for more than a thousand years for its curative properties.

### Parts used

Inner bark.

### Active constituents

The main active ingredient in this plant are the 18 quinones, the main ones being the naphthoquinones, of which lapachol and a form of lapachone are two of the most important. Other constituents are lapachenole, the bioflavonoid quercetin, carnosol, indoles, coenzyme Q, alkaloids and steroidal saponins.

### How it works in the body

Lapachol was isolated as early as 1882, and in 1956 its antibacterial action was confirmed by research in Brazil which established Pao d'Arco as a valuable natural antibiotic. Further tests showed derivatives of this constituent also had antifungal properties effective against ringworm, vaginal thrush, and gastrointestinal candidiasis. Carnosol is a strong antioxidant which mops up free radicals in the body, and is thought to be responsible for the reputation of Pao d'Arco as an anticarcinogenic. In addition, the indoles have been identified as being active in detoxifying the body from carcinogens. A form of lapachone has an antiviral action, which has been used against viruses such as herpes simplex and polio, and also against retroviruses, which are particularly implicated in cancer, especially leukemia, and AIDS. Pao d'Arco also demonstrates activity against some tropical parasites, and the alkaloids show some evidence of benefit in diabetes. Its detoxifying element is useful in skin complaints, and its anti-inflammatory action for conditions such as cystitis, prostatitis and intestinal inflammation.

### Applications

As a decoction, drink 200 ml (8 fl oz), three times a day. As a tincture, take 3 ml (60 drops), three times a day. For vaginal thrush, soak a tampon in a strong infusion of the herb and insert as usual, in addition to taking the herb orally. Tablets are available commercially.

### Indications

- Bacterial and viral infection, especially ear, nose, and throat.
- Fungal problems, including vaginal thrush and candidiasis of the gastrointestinal tract.
- Cancer and leukemia, in addition to orthodox treatments.
- Inflammatory conditions, including cystitis, prostatitis and intestinal inflammation.
- HIV, AIDS, chronic fatigue syndrome and other immune-related illnesses.
- Flu and colds.

*141*

# DANDELION

*Compositae* TARAXACUM OFFICINALE (*pu gong ying*)

Chinese pharmaceutical name: *herba taraxaci mongolici cum radice*

The shiny leaves of this plant are noted for their jagged, tooth-like shape; in fact, it derives its common name from the French *dent de lion*, lion's tooth. This well-known weed, with its bright yellow flowers, is found on wasteland and in cultivated areas. It originated in Europe and Asia, but now grows worldwide.

### History

The botanical name comes from the Greek *taraxos*, meaning disorder, and *aka*, meaning remedy.

### Parts used

Leaves and root.

### Active constituents

Sesquiterpene lactones, triterpenes, phenolic acids, polysaccharides, carotenoids, vitamins A and C and potassium.

### How it works in the body

The leaves contain a large quantity of potassium, which balances their function as a powerful diuretic. This is in contrast to orthodox diuretics, which need a potassium supplement to balance the requirements of the body. In Chinese terms, this herb resolves painful urinary ailments. The root acts differently and is used to improve the function of the liver and as a mild laxative. In Chinese usage, dandelion is indicated for heat disorders, especially in the liver; where the eyes are red, swollen and painful; and for damp-heat jaundice. Both leaf and root act as a tonic to the gallbladder. The herb's detoxifying properties are thought to be beneficial in removing the effects of pollution on the body. In addition, the Chinese use it internally and topically where there are firm or hard abscesses, especially of the breast and digestive system. In women who are breastfeeding, it promotes lactation. The Chinese properties are bitter, sweet and cold.

### Applications

Use fresh in salads or soups. Include in tonic wines to cleanse the system and eliminate toxins; take one sherryglassful a day. Use the leaf as an infusion, taking 200 ml (8 fl oz) three times daily for water retention. Also use the leaf as a tincture, 2 ml (40 drops), three times a day. The root is prepared as a decoction. Take 200 ml (8 fl oz), twice a day. As a tincture, the root can be taken, 2 ml (40 drops), three times a day. The Chinese dosage is 9–30 g (½–1½ oz).

### Indications

- **The leaf** in cases of water retention, e.g. in high blood pressure. Also to promote removal of waste products by the kidneys, e.g. in arthritic conditions.
- **The root** as a tonic to the liver, especially in arthritic conditions to improve removal of toxins, and in skin complaints such as eczema, psoriasis and acne. Also as a gentle laxative. It has a bitter taste and, taken before a meal, helps to stimulate appetite.
- **The leaf and root** as a gallbladder tonic, especially where there are gallstones.
- **As a detoxifier** where there has been undue strain on the body, e.g. excess alcohol consumption.

### Contraindications

As the bitter effect has a stimulating action on the digestion, take this remedy after meals for excess acid or stomach ulcers. The Chinese caution that over-dosage can cause mild diarrhoea.

# THYME
*Labiatae* THYMUS VULGARIS

Common, or garden, thyme is a native of the Mediterranean region, while wild thyme is native to Britain and Europe. It is used similarly to common thyme, which is a shrub with pinkish purple flowers that grows to around 30 cm (1 ft). A huge number of species of thyme is now cultivated in many parts of the world.

### History
The botanical name *Thymus* probably comes from a Greek word meaning to make a burnt offering or fumigate, most likely due to its use as an incense and as an antiseptic. It is also suggested that it may derive from the Greek *thumus*, meaning courage, and in medieval England, thyme was embroidered on tokens given to knights to enhance their valour in battle. The honey from bees that feed on thyme is highly praised, and the Romans used it to flavour cheese and liqueurs; thyme is still widely used to flavour food today. Culpeper said of thyme that it was 'a noble strengthener of the lungs, as notable a one as grows, neither is there scarce a better remedy growing for that disease in children which they commonly called the chin-cough (whooping cough).'

### Parts used
Whole herb, essential oil.

### Active constituents
Volatile oil, especially thymol, with cineole, borneol and others, flavonoids, caffeic acid and tannins.

### How it works in the body
As Culpeper suggested, thyme is primarily a remedy for the respiratory system. The thymol is responsible for its expectorant and antiseptic qualities, which are invaluable for treating chest infections and other respiratory ailments. In the urinary tract system, thymol is beneficial as an antiseptic. The thymol acts with other constituents as an antispasmodic, and this has a sedative effect which is particularly valuable in children's asthma and for those who suffer from hayfever. In addition, there is an antilarval action. In the musculoskeletal system, the oil can be used topically in a base oil as a counterirritant, that is, to draw blood to an area and to warm a cold joint in cases of rheumatic disorder.

### Applications
As an infusion, take 200 ml (8 fl oz), twice a day. As tincture, take 2 ml (40 drops), three times daily. As a syrup, thyme combined with liquorice can be taken for coughs and sore throats, 10 ml (2 tsp), three times a day. The essential oil may be used alone, or with others, in a base oil, 2 drops in 50 ml (4 tbsp), as a rub to stimulate circulation and warm cold joints. When added to water, the essential oil may also be used as an inhalation to ease tight airways. Add the infusion to the bath to relax tired and aching muscles.

### Indications
- Respiratory complaints, such as asthma, bronchitis, hayfever, sore throats and coughs.
- Arthritic complaints where there are cold joints.
- Tired and aching muscles.
- Urinary tract infections (in combination with other herbs).
- Worms.

### Contraindications
**Do not** take more than the stated dosage. **Do not** take the essential oil internally. **Do not** use the oil externally during pregnancy.

# LIMEBLOSSOM

*Tiliaceae* TILIA EUROPAEA

Limeblossom, or limeflower as it is also known, is a tree that grows to a height of 30 m (100 ft). It has bright green heart-shaped leaves and yellowish white flowers which hang in clusters. It comes originally from Europe, but there is a species that grows in North America, *Tilia americana*, which has similar properties.

### History

The light-coloured wood is easy to work and is often used for carvings and furniture. Lime honey from the flowers is regarded as one of the most delicately flavoured. In many of the old herbals, limeblossoms were claimed to have a sedative, antispasmodic effect in cases of epilepsy, and it was thought that if a patient were laid under the tree, it would help to reduce the severity of a seizure. Limes are often planted as street trees and they are blamed for the sticky black substance that drops on to pavements and parked cars. This is, in fact, due to a parasite which lives on the tree, rather than a secretion from the tree itself. The North American species, commonly called basswood, was, according to Vogel, used by forest Indians for treating burns.

### Parts used

Flowers.

### Active constituents

Volatile oil, flavonoids, mucilage, phenolic acids, tannins.

### How it works in the body

The relaxing qualities of limeblossom make it extremely useful in the nervous system, where it has applications for conditions requiring an antispasmodic action, for example, in cases of stress and tension. It is helpful as a remedy for sleeplessness due to its sedative action. For headaches, especially those caused by excess catarrh, this is an excellent remedy. In the cardiovascular system, limeblossom is used to treat high blood pressure, and it has a reputation for helping to lower cholesterol associated with arteriosclerosis. In the digestive system it is used for indigestion associated with nervous tension. It also has a diaphoretic action, which helps the body to sweat out toxins. This, combined with its anticatarrhal properties, makes it helpful in treating colds and flu.

### Applications

As an infusion, use 200 ml (8 fl oz), three times a day for indigestion, stress, headaches and general tension. Use the infusion in the bath to calm and relax. Take 2½–5 ml (½–1 tsp) of the tincture at bedtime for sleeplessness. Take 2 ml (40 drops) three times a day for high blood pressure.

### Indications

- Indigestion and stress-related stomach complaints.
- Insomnia.
- Headaches, especially where there is excess catarrh.
- Symptoms of colds and flu.
- High blood pressure, to lower cholesterol levels.

### Contraindications

**Do not** use this herb in cases of low blood pressure.

# COLTSFOOT

*Compositae* TUSSILAGO FARFARA *(kuan dong hua)*

This common plant originated in Europe and Asia and is now found extensively in North America. The broad green leaves are heart-shaped and the stems are topped with star-like, yellow flowers.

### History

Coltsfoot's botanical name, *Tussilago farfara* indicates its usage: *tussive* means cough and *farfara*, to go – in other words, dispels coughs. Another name was *Filius ante patrem* or 'the son before the father' because the flowers appear first, then die off before the leaves grow. The herb has long been a symbol of herbal medicine and has enjoyed a reputation as a remedy for lung problems, including asthma and bronchitis, as it was included in a mixture of herbs that was smoked. Sticks of coltsfoot rock are still sold for the relief of coughs. In China the flowers are preferred, while in Europe the leaves are used exclusively, since it is thought there is a higher proportion of toxic constituents in the flowers.

### Parts used

Leaves.

### Active constituents

Flavonoids, mucilage (about 8 per cent, consisting mainly of poly-saccharides), pyrrolizidine alkaloids, tannin.

### How it works in the body

The flavonoids have an anti-spasmodic and anti-inflammatory effect, which eases spasm in the lungs during asthma and bronchitis attacks, allowing easier breathing. The polysaccharides are anti-inflammatory, which helps to calm irritated lung tissue, and they also act as an expectorant for excess phlegm and mucus. These constituents work together to improve the immune system and to promote a healthy respiratory system. The pyrrolizidine alkaloids are thought to be harmful to the liver, but they are largely destroyed when coltsfoot is prepared as a decoction.

### Applications

The herb is used as a decoction for the treatment of coughs and other chest complaints. It is combined with other herbs as a tobacco in herbal cigarettes to relieve spasm in asthma and bronchitis. As a tincture, take 1 ml (20 drops) twice daily to improve the lungs. It is particularly good for coughs when used as a syrup. The Chinese dosage is 1.5–9 g ($\frac{1}{16}$–½ oz).

### Indications

• Dry and irritating coughs.
• To improve the general health of the lungs where there are complaints, such as asthma and bronchitis.

### Contraindications

**Do not** use for longer than one month at a time. Use only the leaves, not the flowers. **Do not** take while pregnant or breastfeeding. **Do not** give to children under six years old.

---

### Benefits of coltsfoot

Helps to strengthen lungs

Eases dry and irritating coughs

# STINGING NETTLE

*Urticaceae* URTICA DIOICA

A familiar plant on wasteground, stinging nettle is found in many parts of the world. It reaches a height of about 1.2 m (4 ft) and has serrated green leaves and flowers that grow in clusters around the stem. Male and female flowers are sometimes found on the same plant, but more usually they appear on different plants. The main feature of the nettle is the fine stinging hairs that cover both leaves and stem.

### History

The plant's botanical name comes from the Latin *uro*, I burn, a reference to the stinging nature of the plant, and *dioica*, two houses, which refers to the male and female plants being separate. The common name, nettle, comes from the Old English word *noedl* or needle. The stinging nettle was said to have been introduced into Britain by the Romans, who rubbed it on their joints in the belief that the stinging encouraged blood to flow the area, and helped to offset the effects of Britain's damp, cold climate. It was also taken, along with the other first herbs of spring, as a tonic. Nettle has been used for many purposes, for example the tough fibres were woven into cloth. This property of the plant was immortalized in Hans Christian Andersen's story of a princess who had to weave cloaks of nettle for eleven brothers who had been turned into swans, in order to give them back their human form. Nettle has also been used to make paper. In 1835, acting on the advice of Native Americans, Vogel found that he was able to cure his patients of scurvy by using nettle.

### Parts used

Herb and root.

### Active constituents

Chlorophyll, indoles (e.g. histamine and serotonin), acetylcholine, vitamin C, iron and dietary fibre.

### How it works in the body

Although the growing nettle stings externally, it has no such effect when it has been subjected to heat, either by cooking it or making it into an infusion. Ironically, it acts as an anti-allergenic in skin complaints and, taken internally, can be used to treat eczema and related allergies. It is also antihemorrhagic and acts as an astringent to stop excessive bleeding, either from wounds or in the reproductive system to diminish heavy menstrual bleeding. The vitamin C and iron content make it an excellent tonic for anaemia. The root has been used in the treatment of enlarged prostate glands.

### Applications

As an infusion, take 200 ml (8 fl oz), twice daily; as a decoction of the roots, take 200 ml (8 fl oz) daily. As a tincture, take 3 ml (60 drops), three times a day. The young top leaves, picked in spring, can be made into a soup which can be taken daily as a tonic.

### Indications

- Skin conditions, such as eczema.
- Allergic conditions, including hayfever and asthma.
- Iron tonic.
- In the reproductive system to ease heavy bleeding.
- Enlargement of the prostate gland (root).

### Contraindications

A small number of people find that nettle causes irritation; if this occurs, discontinue use.

# VALERIAN

*Valerianaceae* VALERIANA OFFICINALIS

This plant is native to Europe and Asia and has become naturalized in North America. Valerian grows to about 1 m (3 ft) high and, since it flourishes in wet, marshy conditions, it is often found near rivers. The leaves occur in pairs and the flowers are pale pink or white, with a distinctive smell.

### History

The name is thought to come from the Latin *valere*, meaning health. Dioscorides and Galen named the plant *phu*, a reference to its rather unpleasant odour.

It is this very feature which is thought to make valerian so attractive to both rats and cats: it is suggested that the Pied Piper of Hamlyn had a supply of the herb in his pockets with which he lured the rats out of the town. It known as a herbal remedy in Anglo-Saxon times, and was employed as a treatment for epilepsy in medieval England, when it was given the name 'all heal'. Traditionally, valerian been used as a treatment for over-stimulation of the nervous system. During the First World War it was used in England for shellshock. According to Vogel, the Incas used valerian, together with sea algae, as an unguent for massage.

### Parts used

Root.

### Active constituents

Volatile oil containing valerenic acid, iridoids known as valepotriates, alkaloids, flavonoids, sterols and tannins.

### How it works in the body

Valerian's usefulness in the nervous system is mainly due to the valepotriates, which have a sedative effect on the brain. One of its main uses is in insomnia, where it both helps sufferers to fall asleep more quickly and allows them to wake in the morning without feeling stupefied. It is particularly valuable for those whose minds are so active they cannot switch off enough to relax. It is helpful for all types of stress-related anxiety, since it does not impair the ability to concentrate, but has a calming effect. It is also useful in treating numerous other ailments, for example, digestive complaints where there is a contributing stress or tension factor. It is also a muscle relaxant, and is used, with other herbs, in the cardiovascular system to treat high blood pressure.

### Applications

As a decoction, take 100 ml (4 fl oz), twice daily. For insomnia, take 200 ml (8 fl oz), at night. The tincture may be taken, 2 ml (40 drops), three times a day. Tablets are available commercially.

### Indications

- Insomnia, especially where the mind is overactive.
- Stress and anxiety, for short periods.
- Digestive complaints where stress is a factor, in combination with other herbs.
- High blood pressure, in combination with other herbs.

### Contraindications

In rare instances, people find this herb more stimulating than relaxing. If this is the case, discontinue use.

# CRAMPBARK
*Caprifoliaceae* VIBURNUM OPULUS/PRUNIFOLIUM

Crampbark, or guelder rose as it is sometimes known, is native to both North America and Europe. It is a shrub, belonging to the same family as the elder tree, and grows to a height of approximately 3 m (9 ft). It is commonly found in woodland and hedges.

### History

The name guelder rose comes from a province in Holland where the plant was first cultivated. Native Americans, including the Ojibwas and Meskwakis, traditionally used the remedy for cramping conditions. The plant has been included in the US National Formulary as an antispasmodic and sedative and for the treatment of asthma.

### Parts used

Bark from branches – only small quantities may be harvested at any one time, since the wholesale removal of large amounts of bark could kill the tree.

### Active constituents

Hydroquinones, coumarins, tannins.

### How it works in the body

Crampbark acts as a muscle relaxant, particularly of smooth muscle. As a spasmolytic, *Viburnum opulus* acts on the body tissues as a whole, while *V. prunifolium* is more specific in its action on the uterus. For this reason its main function has to do with the reproductive system, for example, to relieve the cramping that occurs during a menstrual period. It is also effective in cases of threatened miscarriage, but should only be used in this context under the supervision of a qualified herbal or medical practitioner. In addition, it has uses in many other systems of the body: in the stomach to relieve symptoms in conditions such as irritable bowel syndrome; in the respiratory system to help relax the airways in asthma; and for the musculoskeletal system to relieve the tension of arthritic pain. It is also employed in the cardiovascular system, together with other herbs, to help reduce high blood pressure.

### Applications

For internal use as a decoction, the herb is taken when spasm is present, rather than on a continuous basis. To relieve cramp from a period or other cause, take 100 ml (4 fl oz), up to a maximum of six times daily. The tincture can be similarly used; take 2½ ml (50 drops), up to six times daily. For external relief of muscle spasm, add 2 ml (40 drops) of the tincture to 30 g (1½ oz) of a cream such as comfrey, and mix well in. The addition of 2 ml (40 drops) of lobelia tincture to this will enhance the anti-spasmodic effect. Apply up to three times a day.

### Indications

- Relief of uterine and ovarian pain and cramping.
- In cases of threatened miscarriage, only under the supervision of a herbal or medical practitioner.
- Cramping of the muscles due to arthritic conditions.
- Muscle tension and spasm due to stress or night cramps.
- High blood pressure.
- Asthma.

### Contraindications

**Do not** take this remedy during pregnancy. **Do not** take it when low blood pressure is present.

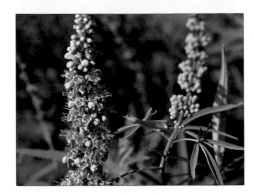

# CHASTE BERRY

*Verbenaceae* VITEX AGNUS CASTUS

Chaste berry is a native of the Mediterranean regions. It is a small tree which grows to about 7 m (21 ft) in height. The leaves, with five to seven leaflets, are dark green above and grey beneath; the spikes of small purple flowers have an aromatic fragrance and give way to dark purple berries in the autumn.

### History

In evidence of the age-old use of the herb both as a promoter of chastity and fertility in women, Athenian women were said to strew their couches with chaste berry in ceremonial rites connected with Demeter, the ancient Greek goddess of agricultural fertility and the protector of marriage and women. At the same time, chaste berry has been used to lower the libido in men, and in Italy it is ceremonially cast in the path of male novices when they first enter monasteries, hence its common name of monk's pepper. At other times it has been used to relieve paralysis, general weakness and pain in the limbs.

### Parts used

Berries.

### Active constituents

Iridoid glycosides (including aucibin and agnoside), volatile oil (cineol), fixed oils, alkaloids (viticine) and flavonoids (casticin).

### How it works in the body

Chaste berry has distinct actions, depending on whether it is given to men or women. Commonly used as a woman's herb, it affects the pituitary gland, which sends chemical messages to regulate the hormone balance in the body. It is thought to regulate the two main hormones, oestrogen and progesterone, and is invaluable in treating many disorders in the reproductive system that are due to an imbalance of these hormones, for example, PMS, irregular periods and infertility. It can also be used to treat acne, which is a result of hormonal imbalance at puberty or menopause. For men, the herb acts to depress the male androgen hormones, which are responsible for, among other things, the male sex drive. For this reason the herb is only rarely given to men.

### Applications

The tincture should be taken in water first thing in the morning, 1 ml (20 drops), increasing to 2 ml (40 drops) if needed, daily. Tablets are available commercially. To enjoy the full benefit from this remedy, it should be taken for at least three months.

### Indications

- For conditions where there is hormonal imbalance.
- PMS (mood swings, bloating, tenderness of the breasts).
- Irregular periods.
- Migraine associated with the menstrual cycle.
- Acne associated with the menstrual cycle.
- Acne associated with puberty or the menopause.
- Infertility.

### Contraindications

Do **not** exceed the stated dosage. This herb has been shown to work at these levels and it is not advisable to increase the amounts taken. If in any doubt, consult a qualified herbal practitioner.

# MAIZE (CORNSILK)

*Gramineae* ZEA MAYS *(yu mi xu)*

Although it originated in South America, maize is now grown worldwide, wherever the climate is sufficiently warm. It is a grass which grows to about 3 m (10 ft) high and produces large cobs of edible grains. The name cornsilk refers to the threadlike silky tassel that emerges from the top of the female flower when it is ready for pollination.

### History

Maize is primarily a foodstuff, so the medicinal part – the 'silks' – is usually discarded. It has long been used medicinally by Native Americans, usually as a poultice for skin conditions. European pioneers found it a useful diuretic and remedy for cystitis. Chinese research has found evidence of its value in the circulatory system as an agent to lower blood pressure and reduce blood-clotting time.

### Parts used

Cornmeal (kernels) externally, cornsilk internally.

### Active constituents

Saponins, allantoin, sterols, alkaloid (hordenine), mucilage, vitamins C and K and potassium.

### How it works in the body

This plant works mainly in the urinary tract. The saponins act largely as an anti-inflammatory in the body and the allantoin as a healing agent, the mucilage having a soothing effect on irritated tissues. The potassium balances out the diuretic effect of the herb, when it is used in conditions of water retention and other urinary tract conditions such as cystitis and prostatitis. Vitamin K is a fat-soluble vitamin essential for blood clotting within the body.

### Applications

Use cornsilk as an infusion, fresh or dried. In urinary tract infections, take 1 cup, 200 ml (8 fl oz), three times a day. Use a decoction of the meal as a poultice for wounds and sores. As a tincture, take 3 ml (50 drops), three times a day for conditions such as cystitis. The Chinese dosage is 15–30 g (¼–1½ oz).

### Indications

- To reduce water retention, for example in high blood pressure.
- Frequent urination, e.g., cystitis.
- Difficulty in passing water, e.g., prostatitis.
- For kidney problems, e.g., kidney stones.

### Contraindications

**Do not** take in conditions of low blood pressure.

---

**Benefits of cornsilk**

*Eases symptoms of prostatitis*

*Helpful in kidney disorders*

*Helps lower blood pressure*

*Soothes irritation in cystitis*

# GINGER

*Zingiberaceae* ZINGIBER OFFICINALE *(sheng jiang)*

Originally from Asia, ginger is now grown in many other tropical countries, including parts of China, North America, Jamaica and Africa. The aerial part of the plant consists of a green stalk with narrow leaves and a spike of yellow or white flowers. It is the root or rhizome, with its long, tuberous joints, that is used in cooking. The plant must be a year old before the root can be used.

### History

Ginger is said to have been employed since Greek and Roman times for its medicinal benefits, and it was the Romans who introduced this plant into Britain. Research continues into the benefits of ginger, with recent studies confirming its use as an anti-emetic, and also its value in the treatment of bacillary dysentry.

### Parts used

Root or rhizome.

### Active constituents

Volatile oil, phenolic compounds, including gingerols and shogaols.

### How it works in the body

The phenolic compounds are the agents responsible for relaxing the muscles of the stomach, and this may also explain their effect in easing travel or motion sickness. Fresh or dried, the root has been shown to minimize vomiting. In addition, the phenolic ingredients act within the stomach as a sedative and painkiller, which helps to reduce over-activity of the gut. In stomach infections, the oil acts as an antiseptic and anti-inflammatory. The gingerols alone are thought to be responsible for ginger's action as a liver protective. In the cardiovascular system, ginger is thought to reduce cholesterol levels, while at the same time increasing a sluggish circulation. In China, the fresh rhizome is used to warm the stomach to ease vomiting and to fight off colds, chills and coughs, especially where there is phlegm, and for bloating. The dried rhizome is used for abdominal pain. The Chinese properties are those of acrid and warm.

### Applications

Take ginger as an infusion, 200 ml (8 fl oz), three times a day to aid digestion or for nausea. For travel sickness, combine it with camomile in a flask and take it before and during a journey. The tincture may be taken, 1 ml (20 drops), three times a day, to improve the circulation and for coughs, colds and flu symptoms. The Chinese dosage indicates 3–9 g (⅛–½ oz).

### Indications

- Travel and motion sickness.
- Indigestion and nausea; sickness in pregnancy.
- Sluggish circulation, especially where hands and feet are cold.
- High cholesterol levels.
- Colds, flu and coughs.
- Over-activity of the gut, wind and bloating.

### Contraindications

In Chinese terms, this herb should **not** be used in cases of lung heat or stomach heat with vomiting. It should be used with caution in lung infections with fevers, or with irritative digestive complaints such as ulcers and acid indigestion.

# ADDITIONAL HERBS

*A brief description of herbs used or mentioned in this book but not listed*

*in the Herbal Directory.*

### Agrimony
*Agrimonia eupatoria* Astringent and tonic properties, making it a valuable remedy for the treatment of childhood diarrhoea and urinary incontinence.

### Arnica
*Arnica montana* One of the best herbs for healing bruising and sprains. **Caution:** *Never take it internally.* Should not be used if the skin is broken.

### Bladderwrack
*Fucus vesiculosus* Very useful in regulating the thyroid. Helps an under-active thyroid and goiter.

### Boneset
*Eupatorium perfoliatum* One of the best remedies for the relief of symptoms associated with flu – relieves fevers, catarrh, aches and pains.

### Borage
*Borago officinalis* Benefits the adrenal glands, helping to restore function after the use of steroids. Also helps boost the immune system.

### Bugleweed
*Lycopus europaeus* Specific use for over-active thyroid, helping with symptoms of palpitations, shaking and difficulty in breathing.

### Catmint
*Nepeta cataria* Traditionally used for the treatment of colds and flu, but also has relaxing and calming properties. Especially suitable for children with fevers.

### Cayenne
*Capsicum minimum* Stimulant and tonic, helping digestive and circulatory disorders. Use in small amounts – approximately one-quarter of recommended general dosage.

### Celery seed
*Apium graveolens* Antiseptic, useful in the treatment of urinary problems and also, with dandelion leaf, in rheumatic conditions.

### Cinnamon
*Cinnamomum zeylanicum* Helps to relieve nausea and vomiting and mild cases of diarrhoea.

### Cloves
*Eugenia caryophyllus* Stimulant to the digestive system. Powerful local antiseptic and mild anesthetic, can also be used for toothache. **Caution:** *Do not swallow the clove pieces.*

### Damiana
*Turnera aphrodisiaca* Helps strengthen the nervous system, and useful as an antidepressant. Strengthens the male reproductive system, thus enhancing libido.

### Elecampane
*Inula helenium* Helpful for treating irritating bronchial coughs, especially in children, and for bronchitis and emphysema. Also helps clear copious catarrh.

### False unicorn root
*Chamaelirium luteum* One of the best tonics for the female reproductive system. Take as a decoction (half a cup, twice daily) or as a tincture (15 drops, twice daily). **Caution:** *Do not exceed the dose, since large amounts may cause nausea or vomiting. Do not take during pregnancy.*

### Fennel
*Foeniculum vulgare* Excellent remedy for colic and flatulence. Helps increase milk flow in breastfeeding.

### Forskolin
*Coleus forskohlii* Used to aid digestion, help reduce blood pressure and improve circulation.

### Golden rod
*Solidago virgaurea* Helpful for coughs, colds and sinusitis. Useful for clearing catarrh in acute and chronic cases.

### Horsetail
*Equisetum arvense* Diuretic and astringent; helpful in the treatment of urinary disorders, including bedwetting and incontinence.

### Hyssop

*Hyssopus officinalis* Helps relieve coughs and colds. Also a relaxant for anxiety and hysteria.

### Juniper berries

*Juniperus communis* Excellent remedy for cystitis. Also used externally as an oil to ease painful muscles and joints. **Caution:** *Do not take in pregnancy or with kidney disease.*

### Milk thistle

*Silybum marianum* Also known as Our Lady's Milk Thistle, Blessed Thistle and Holy Thistle. Aid to the liver, helping to promote the flow of bile. Excellent remedy to promote milk flow when breastfeeding.

### Myrrh

*Commiphora molmol* Strong anti-microbial action used for the treatment of infections, particularly as mouthwash.

### Pilewort

*Ranunculus ficaria* Used specifically to treat haemorrhoids, or piles. Use internally as a tea or externally as an ointment.

### Poke root

*Phytolacca americana* Valuable remedy to clear catarrh and cleanse the lymph system. **Caution:** *In large doses poke root acts as a purgative.*

### Prickly ash bark and berries

*Zanthoxylum americanum* Stimulating tonic for the circulatory system. Helpful for many complaints, such as poor circulation, varicose veins and cramps.

### Raspberry leaves

*Rubus ideaus* Toning for the womb. **Caution:** *Use only during the last three months of pregnancy.*

### Red clover

*Trifolium pratense* Useful remedy for childhood eczema and hyperactivity; helps to cleanse the system.

### Slippery elm

*Ulmus fulva* Soothing herb for digestive complaints. Take as decoction, using one part powder to eight parts water, or as pills. Also used externally as a poultice to treat boils and abscesses.

### Stone root

*Collinsonia canadensis* Mainly used in the treatment of stones or gravel in the urinary system and the gallbladder.

### Tea tree

*Melaleuca alternifolia* Used for its antiseptic and antifungal properties. **Caution:** *Can irritate the skin, so use in a carrier/base oil for athlete's foot and insect bites.*

### Thuja

*Thuja occidentalis* Used externally to treat warts and fungal infections. **Caution:** *Use internally only under professional supervision.*

### Vervain

*Verbena officinalis* Nervine tonic that will strengthen the nervous system while relaxing and easing tension. Useful for depression following influenza.

### Wild oats

*Avena sativa* Bridge between food and medicine. Useful as general tonic for the nervous system, especially in cases of debility or exhaustion. Antidepressant. Take as gruel, porridge or tincture.

### Wild yam

*Dioscorea villosa* Valuable herb that has antispasmodic, anti-inflammatory, and antirheumatic properties, as well as many properties found in the contraceptive pill. Used for colic, painful periods and arthritis.

# KITCHEN REMEDIES

Basic ingredients found in nearly every kitchen can be used as herbal remedies. Listed below are some common ailments and the kitchen remedies that can be used to treat them gently and effectively.

### COLDS AND FLU

To make a warming drink, combine 5 ml (1 tsp) lemon juice with one crushed clove of garlic, a table-spoon of honey, and a pinch of either powdered cinnamon or ginger, and pour on a cupful of hot water. The lemon juice is antiseptic and contains vitamin C to fight off a cold; the garlic is antibiotic, helps reduce catarrh and is effective against all kinds of infections; while the cinnamon and ginger are warming.

### TOOTHACHE

To ease an aching tooth until you can see a dentist, hold a clove in your mouth over the tooth and slowly nibble away at it. You should not use more than two cloves at any one time, and should not swallow the pieces. If you have clove oil, put one or two drops on a small piece of cotton-wool and hold it over the tooth to obtain relief. Repeat twice if needed. Cloves are both anti-septic and pain-killing.

### ITCHING
### SKIN/ECZEMA

Ordinary porridge oats can be used to alleviate itching skin and heal eczema. Prepare a decoction of the oats, strain and add the liquid to a lukewarm bath (*see* Herbal Methods section). Externally, oats are

soothing and healing to the skin as well as cleansing. Taken as porridge or as a juice, oats are nutritious and strengthen the nervous system, acting as an antidepressant, and also helping to reduce cholesterol.

### COUGHS AND SORE
### THROATS

Take half an onion, sliced, and alternate with sugar in layers on a plate. Place a bowl over this and leave overnight before pouring off the juice, which makes an excellent cough syrup. Onions are both antiseptic and healing.

### DIARRHOEA

A simple but effective emergency treatment is to drink a cup of ordinary tea without milk or sugar. The tannins will coat the lining of the stomach and act as an astringent, relieving the symptoms. For children, dilute fresh lemon juice with water and add a little honey. If the condition persists, you must seek additional help since you run the risk of dehydrating, which is potentially very serious.

### STINGS AND BITES

To alleviate the pain from insect stings and bites, use cold cider vinegar as a wash. To prevent insect bites, especially before going away on holiday, eat plenty of garlic, since it will dissuade insects from bothering you.

# A FAMILY REMEDY CHEST

A home herbal medicine chest can be prepared in addition to a conventional first-aid kit, but should not replace it. (A conventional kit will contain such necessities as bandages, scissors, and thermometer.) The essentials can be supplemented by a range of herbal remedies which will enhance your family's well-being.

### OBTAINING YOUR REMEDIES

Some of the remedies will be available commercially. Others may be obtained by using the Herbal Methods section (*see* pp.14–31) to prepare the ointments, creams, etc. that will be useful for you and your family. Refer to the Herbal Directory (*see* pp.100–151) for information on individual herbs and their dosages, or refer to the general dosages information in the Herbal Methods section (*see* p.16). Commercial remedies will always state recommended dosage.

## PILLS

### SLIPPERY ELM

A useful remedy, which will ease diarrhea and gastric upsets. Also available as a powder.

### ECHINACEA

Invaluable for infections; antiviral and antibacterial.

## CAPSULES

### GARLIC OIL

Use to combat infections. Take before and during a vacation to deter insects from biting. For ear infections, open the capsule, place two drops on a small piece of cottonwool and place it in the ear.

## CREAMS

### ARNICA

Use for bruises and sprains. Do not apply to broken skin. Discontinue when discoloration disappears.

### COMFREY

Use on the skin area over sprains, strains and fractures. Do not apply to broken skin.

## OINTMENTS

### MARIGOLD

Use for cuts and grazes. Ideal for children, and may be used for diaper rash to protect baby's skin.

## ESSENTIAL OILS

### LAVENDER

Apply to mild burns after cooling for 10 minutes. Acts as painkiller. Use neat on insect bites and stings. *See* Herbal Directory (p.125) for its many other uses.

### THYME

Use as inhalation (*see* Herbal Methods, p.24) to ease breathing, catarrh or sinusitis. Add five drops to a bath to relieve tired and aching muscles.

## GEL

### ALOE VERA

Use gel or keep the fresh plant on hand and break off a leaf when needed. Heals cuts and scrapes. Good for sunburn and itchy skin.

## HERBS

Which herbs you keep on hand will be entirely a matter of personal choice. However, some suggestions might be, camomile to calm digestive upsets and aid sleep; elderflower for treating colds and flu, hayfever, etc.; limeblossom in cases of poor sleep and shock; meadowsweet for an acid stomach, arthritic pains and headaches; nettle to treat allergies and heavy bleeding.

# GLOSSARY

*A brief description of some of the terms used in this book.*

**Alterative**
Acts as a blood cleanser.

**Anodyne**
Pain killer.

**Antiallergenic**
Helps reduce allergic reactions.

**Antibacterial**
Works against bacteria which cause infection.

**Anticarcinogenic**
Works against cancer.

**Anticatarrhal**
Reduces excess catarrh.

**Anticholesterol**
Reduces cholesterol levels.

**Antidepressant**
Active against depression.

**Antiemetic**
Helps prevent vomiting.

**Antifungal**
Works against fungal infections.

**Antihaemorrhagic**
Helps prevent bleeding.

**Anti-inflammatory**
Reduces inflammation.

**Antioxidant**
Helps prevent the breakdown of tissues.

**Antispasmodic**
Reduces muscle spasm.

**Antithrombotic**
Reduces blood clotting levels.

**Antiviral**
Works against viruses which cause infection.

**Antiseptic**
Helps prevent infection.

**Astringent**
Coats the surface of the skin, reducing fluids and bleeding.

**Carminative**
Helps relieve indigestion.

**Counterirritant**
Causes local irritation by drawing blood, thus acting as pain-reliever.

**Decongestant**
Eases congestion caused by excess mucus.

**Demulcent**
Coats the surface, soothing and aiding healing.

**Diaphoretic**
Encourages the removal of toxins through sweating.

**Diuretic**
Helps relieve water retention by encouraging urination.

**Emmenagogue**
Encourages menstruation by stimulating uterine muscles.

**Emollient**
Soothing to the skin.

**Expectorant**
Promotes the cough reflex, aiding the expulsion of phlegm.

**Exudate**
Discharge from sore or wound.

**Haemostatic**
Reduces bleeding.

**Hyperthyroid**
Over-activity of the thyroid gland.

**Hypoglycemic**
Reduces blood sugar levels.

**Laxative**
Promotes mild bowel evacuation.

**Mucilage**
Gelatinous, demulcent, and soothing.

**Neuralgia**
Nerve pain or irritation.

**Oedema**
Swelling of the tissues due to excess water retention.

**Purgative**
Promotes strong evacuation of the bowels.

**Refrigerant**
Cooling and pain-relieving.

**Relaxant**
Relaxes muscles.

**Sedative**
Reduces the activity of the nervous system.

**Soporific**
Causes drowsiness or sleep.

**Tonic**
Re-balances and nourishes the system.

**Topically**
External use.

**Vulnary**
Wound-healer.

# FURTHER READING AND USEFUL ADDRESSES

## Books

Bensky, D. and Barlott, R. *Chinese Herbal Medicine – Formulas and Strategies*. Eastland Press. Washington D.C., 1990.

Chevallier, A. *The Encyclopedia of Medicinal Plants*. Dorling Kindersley. London, 1996.

Curtis, S. Fraser, R. and Kohler, I. *Neal's Yard Natural Remedies*. Arkana. London, 1988.

Fratkin, J. *Chinese Herbal Patent Formulas*. Institute for Traditional Medicine. Portland, Oregon.

Fratkin, J. *Herbal Patent Formulas: A Practical Guide*. Institute for Traditional Medicine. Portland, Oregon, 1986.

Grieve, M. *A Modern Herbal*. Penguin Books. London, 1989.

Hoffman, D. *The Holistic Herbal*. Element Books. Dorset, 1983.

Lust, J. *The Herb Book*. Bantam. New York, 1986.

McIntyre, A. *The Herbal for Mother and Child*. Element Books. Dorset, 1992.

McIntyre, A. *Herbs for Common Ailments*. Gaia Books. London, 1992.

Ody, P. *The Complete Medicinal Herbal*. Dorling Kindersley. London, 1993.

Vogel, V. *American Indian Medicine*. University of Oklahoma Press, 1970.

Wren, R. C. *Potter's New Cyclopaedia of Botanical Drugs and Preparations*. C. W. Daniel Company Ltd. Saffron Walden, Essex, 1988.

## Other publications

*The Canadian Journal of Herbalism*. 11 Winthrop Place, Stoney Creek, Ontario, L8G 3M3, Canada.

*European Journal of Herbal Medicine*. National Institute of Medical Herbalists, 56 Longbrook Street, Exeter, Devon EX4 6AH, England.

## Where to find a qualified practitioner

The National Institute of Medical Herbalists (est. 1864), 56 Longbrook Street, Exeter, Devon EX4 6AH, England.

The General Council and Register of Consultant Herbalists, 18 Sussex Square, Brighton, East Sussex BN2 5AA, England.

Ontario Herbalists Association, 7 Alpine Avenue, Toronto, Ontario M6P 3R6, Canada.

American Holistic Medical Association, 6728 Old McLean Village Drive, McLean, VA 22101, USA.

American Herbalist Guild, PO Box 1683, Soquel, CA 95073, USA.

National Herbalists Association of Australia, Suite 305, BST House, 3 Smail Street, Broadway, NSW 2007, Australia.

## Courses

Middlesex University, Queensway, Enfield, Middlesex EN3 4SF, England. Full-time and correspondence courses.

School of Phytotherapy, Bucksteep Manor, Bodle Street Green, Nr Hailsham, East Sussex BN27 4RH, England. Full-time and correspondence courses.

The Dominion Herbal College (est. 1926), 7527 Kingsway, Burnaby, British Columbia V3N 3C1, Canada. Correspondence courses only.

The Canadian School of Phytotherapy (Herbal Medicine), Mohawk College, Hamilton, Ontario, Canada.

National College of Naturopathic Medicine, 11231 S. E. Market St, Portland, OR 97216, USA.

# INDEX

# CREDITS

Quarto would like to acknowledge and thank the following for providing pictures used in this book. While every effort has been made to acknowledge copyright holders we would like to apologize should there have been any omissions.

**Key:** *t*=top  *b*=bottom  *c*=centre  *l*=left  *r*=right

**Pat Brindley** p.104, p.109, p.112, p.116, p.125, p.127, p.130, p.132, p.134; **Julian Cotton** p.69(*b*); **Harry Smith Horticultural Photographic Collection** p.102, p.103, p.105, p.106, p.108, p.110, p.111, p.113, p.115, p.118, p.122, p.124, p.128, p.129, p.133, p.135, p.136, p.138, p.140, p.141, p.142, p.143, p.144, p.145, p.146, p.147, p.148, p.149, p.150, p.151; **The Image Bank** p.24, p.41(*c*), p.52(*b*), p.53(*t*), p.57(*b*), p.62(*b*), p.68(*t*), p.73(*t*), p.75(*t*); **Peter McHoy** p.107, p.114, p.119, p.120, p.121, p.139; **Photos Horticultural Picture Library** p.126; **Photo/Nats Inc.** p.123, p.131, p.137; **Positive Images** p.117; **Pictor International** p.16, p.26, p.39(*tr*), p.61(*b*), p.64(*b*), p.72(*t*), p.78(*b*), p.80(*b*), p.87(*b*), p.95(*t*), p.98(*t*); **Tony Stone Images** p.9, p.11, p.27, p.28, p.41(*b*), p.42(*t*), p.45(*b*), p.47(*b*), p.51(*t*), p.56(*t*), p.63(*t*), p.74(*b*), p.78(*t*), p.79(*t*), p.83(*t*), p.86(*t*), p.90(*l*), p.91(*b*), p.92(*t*), p.93(*b*).

All other photographs are the copyright of Quarto.

Quarto would also like to thank the following for supplying props and equipment for photography:

**Plasterworks** 38 Cross Street, London N1 2BG.

**Neal's Yard Remedies** Neal's Yard, Covent Garden, London WC2.

**East West Herbs Ltd.** 3 Neal's Yard, London WC2.

**Authors' acknowledgements**
This book is dedicated with my dearest love and thanks to Mary for her support, Kelly for her encouragement, and to Megan, who gives me joy and inspiration. **Jade Britton**

To Clive, Ryan and Molly Jo, with thanks for your love and support, and to my beautiful garden. **Tamara Kircher**